Handbook of
Neurological Lists

Handbook of Neurological Lists

Lawrence M. Brass, M.D.
Assistant Professor
Department of Neurology
Yale University School of Medicine
New Haven, Connecticut

Peter K. Stys, M.D., F.R.C.P.(C)
Associate Research Scientist
Department of Neurology
Yale University School of Medicine
New Haven, Connecticut

Churchill Livingstone
New York, Edinburgh, London, Melbourne, Tokyo

Library of Congress Cataloging-in-Publication Data

Brass, Lawrence M.
    Handbook of neurological lists / Lawrence M. Brass, Peter K. Stys.
        p. cm.
    Includes index.
    ISBN 0-443-08696-6
    1. Neurology—Outlines, syllabi, etc.   I. Stys, Peter K.
II. Title.
  [DNLM: 1. Nervous System Diseases—diagnosis—handbooks.
WL 39 B823h]
RC343.6.B73 1991
616.8'0475—dc20
DNLM/DLC
for Library of Congress

© **Churchill Livingstone Inc. 1991**

Distributed in the United Kingdom by Churchill Livingstone, Robert Stevenson House, 1–3 Baxter's Place, Leith Walk, Edinburgh EH1 3AF, and by associated companies, branches, and representatives throughout the world.

Accurate indications, adverse reactions, and dosage schedules for drugs are provided in this book, but it is possible that they may change. The reader is urged to review the package information data of the manufacturers of the medications mentioned.

The Publishers have made every effort to trace the copyright holders for borrowed material. If they have inadvertently overlooked any, they will be pleased to make the necessary arrangements at the first opportunity.

Acquisitions Editor: *Beth Kaufman Barry*
Copy Editor: *Ann Ruzycka*
Production Designer: *Jill Little*
Production Supervisor: *Jeanine Furino*

Printed in the United States of America

First published in 1991   7 6 5 4 3 2 1

To Anna and Lori Ann
for their unfailing encouragement and understanding

Preface

The art and science of neurology is a vast field indeed. Although neurophysiology and clinical neurological diagnosis are amenable to logical thinking and problem-solving, the clinician nevertheless needs to possess a formidable base of seemingly unrelated facts from which to formulate a reasonable plan of diagnosis and management. It is such an assortment of facts that is the most difficult to remember and manipulate.

We set out to write this book not to teach clinical skills nor to discuss the pathophysiology of diseases, but rather to present an organized database of facts in neurology to aid the clinician in systematically approaching a clinical problem. Such facts may be as varied as a compilation of neurotransmitters and their enzymatic pathways, or simply a list of differential diagnoses of muscle disorders. A very convenient way to organize information is by making lists; a hierarchical tree structure, with headings and subheadings, was used to organize facts in a logical manner, in the hope of helping the reader to remember these more easily.

We tried to be as consistent as possible throughout the book. Lists of differential diagnoses for the major disease categories are, for the most part, organized under a familiar template, so that completely different clinical problems can be approached with a common algorithm. The template is organized into eleven major headings, as shown in the Standard Template of Differential Diagnosis, which follows the Contents. Whenever possible, these same headings are repeated for different syndromes, eliminating as much as possible the need to memorize a completely different classification for each syndrome. Thus, whether a patient presents with dystonia or a neuropathy, the same etiological categories of disease should come to mind: vascular, structural, myelin disorders, metabolic disorders, and so on. Such an organization typically begins with the most general and prevalent, and allows the clinician to proceed, with as much detail as he or she requires, to the most rarely encountered disorders. Furthermore, through consistency, the student of neurology will be able to apply this template to syndromes that may not appear in this book, and will thus be able to generate a nearly complete list of differential diagnoses for virtually any case. Of course, not all syndromes can be as readily classified into a standard list of categories; we strayed from the standard classification only when it was necessary to accommodate special diseases or syndromes (for instance, myopathies, by virtue of their distinct etiologies, are better organized under a different classification). Other lists, such as the classification of inherited neurometabolic disorders, are not aimed at etiology, and possess distinct categories.

The lists compiled in this book are by no means complete, but we hope that they will help the student and clinician to approach clinical situations in a more systematic and logical manner. We gratefully acknowledge the contributions of lists, ideas, and suggestions from our colleagues. We would also like to thank those who gave permission to reproduce lists and tables from other sources. Any suggestions for additional lists, or modifications of current ones, for future editions, are most welcome.

Lawrence M. Brass, M.D.
Peter K. Stys, M.D., F.R.C.P. (C)

Contents

Standard Template of Differential Diagnosis

A popular approach to neurological differential diagnosis is to classify diseases by etiology. Although some syndromes are better categorized in other ways, the following list works remarkably well for many diseases encountered in clinical practice. We are first to admit that some disorders, whose pathophysiology is controversial, may not technically belong under their headings (e.g., although migraine is classified under "Vascular," are the transient neurological deficits seen with classical migraine due to vascular effects?), or might just as easily fit under multiple headings (e.g., diabetes is an *endocrine [metabolic]* disorder, commonly presenting as a result of *vascular* compromise). Nevertheless, for the sake of simplicity and consistency, such compromises have been made. Doubtless many disorders will need to be re-classified in the future as our knowledge about pathophysiology becomes more detailed.

Our standard classification consists of eleven headings. These are outlined in some detail in the list "Differential Diagnosis by Etiology." Many of these subheadings (e.g., inherited neurometabolic disorders and CNS vasculitis) have their own more comprehensive classifications elsewhere in this book.

"Vascular" disorders include those that produce neurological deficits as a result of insufficient blood supply to neural tissue. This may be caused by thromboembolism, vasculitis, or a coagulopathy. The "Structural" category includes those causes producing dysfunction solely through mass effect or compression of adjacent tissue. The "Myelin" category describes diseases that result in loss of previously normal myelination, such as multiple sclerosis or postinfectious demyelination, or the production of inherently abnormal myelin as a result of a genetic defect, such as the leukodystrophies.

"Metabolic" disturbances resulting in neurological dysfunction, excluding inherited defects, which are classified under their own heading, encompass a large number of disorders. Five subcategories include diseases of the endocrine system, effects of drugs, exogenous toxins not usually used for medicinal purposes, disorders resulting from nutritional deficiency, and neurological effects resulting from the failure of other organs.

"Infections" are most easily classified according to the causative agent. Additional subcategories (e.g., viruses can be expanded to include RNA, DNA, retroviruses, and slow-viruses) may be created depending on the detail required.

"Neurodegenerative" disorders include a variety of diseases for which a clear cause has not yet been established. "Paraneoplastic" syndromes are those resulting from systemic cancer and not due to structural compression by a tumor mass. These include remote effects, disseminated meningeal spread, and dysfunction mediated by paraproteins.

"Inherited neurometabolic disorders" encompass the many inborn errors of metabolism and genetic and hereditary defects that may present from birth to adulthood. A more comprehensive list of these complex disorders appears elsewhere under its own list.

Many positive and negative signs and symptoms may have an epileptic etiology, and are represented under the "Seizure" heading.

"Trauma," whether mechanical, thermal, electrical, or resulting from ionizing radiation, has its own category.

Finally, "Psychogenic/Psychiatric" cases can present in virtually any form, and always deserve mention in a list of differential diagnoses.

Consider the syndrome of dementia to illustrate how the template organizes information. Vascular causes include multi-infarct dementia. Structural lesions such as chronic subdurals, tumors, or normal pressure hydrocephalus can present with a dementing illness, as can demyelinating diseases such as the leukodystrophies or long-standing cases of multiple sclerosis. Metabolic causes are varied: examples include endocrine disorders such as hypothyroidism or hypercalcemia, drugs such as anticholinergics, toxins such as alcohol or lead, nutritional deficiency (vitamin B_{12}), or failure of renal or hepatic function. Examples of infections presenting with dementia include Creutzfeld-Jakob disease, AIDS dementia, and neurosyphilis. Patients suffering from neurodegenerative disorders such as Alzheimer's or Parkinson's disease or from paraneoplastic syndromes such as limbic encephalitis or meningeal carcinomatosis may exhibit prominent dementia. Many inherited neurometabolic and genetic disorders have dementia as a prominent symptom, as do some chronic and poorly controlled epileptics. CNS trauma may lead to cognitive impairment (dementia pugilistica or "punch-drunk" syndrome), and depression may present with severe cognitive dysfunction. This approach will identify most diseases that need to be ruled out when the clinician is faced with a demented patient.

Abbreviations

·ACTH	adrenocorticotropic hormone
ADH	alcohol dehydrogenase
AIDS	acquired immunodeficiency syndrome
ALS	amyotropic lateral sclerosis
AMI	acute myocardial infarction
A-V	atrioventricular
AVM	arteriovenous malformation
BAL	British anti-lewisite
BCNU	N, N-bis(2-chloroethyl)-N-nitrosourea
cAMP	cyclic adenosine monophosphate
CAT	choline acetyl transferase
CBC	complete blood count
CMV	cytomegalovirus
CN	cranial nerve
CNS	central nervous system
COPD	chronic obstructive pulmonary disease
CP	cerebellopontine
CPEO	chronic progressive external ophthalmoplegia
CPK	creatine phosphokinase
CPT	carnitine palmityl transferase
CSF	cerebrospinal fluid
CT	computed tomography
DDT	dichlorodiphenyltrichloroethane
DIMS	disorders of initiating and maintaining sleep
DOES	disorders of excessive sleep
DST	dexamethasone suppression test
ECHO	enterocytopathogenic human orphan
EEG	electroencephalogram

EKG	electrocardiogram
EMG	electromyogram
EP	evoked potential
ESR	erythrocyte sedimentation rate
FIRD	frontal intermittent rhythmic delta
FSH	follicle-stimulating hormone
GABA	gamma-aminobutyric acid
GABA-T	GABA-transaminase
GANS	granulomatous angiitis of the nervous system
GI	gastrointestinal
GM	monosialoganglioside
Hct	hematocrit
HIV	human immunodeficiency virus
HSMN	hereditary sensorimotor neuropathy
HSN	hereditary sensory neuropathy
HTLV	human T-cell leukemia virus
Ig	immunoglobulin
IM	intramuscular
INH	isoniazid
INO	internuclear ophthalmoplegia
IPSP	inhibitory postsynaptic potential
L-dopa	levodopa
LP	lumbar puncture
LS	lumbosacral
LSD	lysergic acid diethylamide
MADA	myoadenylate deaminase
MAO	monoamine oxidase
MELAS	mitrochondrial myopathy, encephalopathy, lactic acidosis, stroke-like episodes
MERRF	myoclonal epilepsy with red ragged fibers
MI	myocardial infarction
MPTP	1-methyl-4-phenyl-1,2,3,6-tetrahydropyridine
MRI	magnetic resonance imaging

NMJ	neuromuscular junction
OB	oligoclonal bands
OKN	optokinetic nystagmus
PLED	periodic lateralized epileptiform discharges
PME	progressive myoclonus epilepsy
PMH	pure motor hemiparesis
PMN	polymorphonuclear leukocyte
PNS	peripheral nervous system
POSTS	positive occipital sharp transients of sleep
REM	rapid eye movement
SIADH	syndrome of inappropriate antidiuretic hormone
SLE	systemic lupus erythematosus
SREDA	subclinical rhythmic epileptiform discharges of adults
TB	tuberculosis
TIA	transient ischemic attack
TMJ	temporomandibular joint
TRH	thyrotropin-releasing hormone
URI	upper respiratory infection
UTI	urinary tract infection
VA	ventral anterior
VDRL	Venereal Disease Research Laboratory
VL	ventral lateral
VPL	ventral posterolateral
VPM	ventral posteromedial
z-PAM	pralidoxime

1
INTRODUCTORY LISTS

DIFFERENTIAL DIAGNOSIS BY ETIOLOGY

I. Vascular (infarct or hemorrhage, arterial or venous)
   A. Thromboembolism
      1. Atherosclerosis
      2. Thrombus
      3. Cardiogenic emboli
         a. Atrial/mural/valvular thrombus
         b. Bacterial endocarditis
         c. Marantic endocarditis
         d. Atrial myxoma
      4. Paroxysmal embolus
      5. Artery-artery embolus
   B. Small vessel disease
   C. Migraine
   D. Vasculitis/connective tissue disease
   E. Dessection/dysplasia/vasospasm
   F. Hemorrhage (e.g., subarachnoid hemorrhage)
   G. Hematomas (discussed under Structural)
   H. Blood as primary disorder
      1. Coagulopathy (birth control pill, pregnancy, anticoagulants)
      2. Hyperviscosity (paraproteinemias, leukemia, polycythemia, sickle cell disease)

II. Structural (compression from mass effect or structural defect)
   A. Tumor
      1. Neoplasm
         a. Primary
            (1) Astrocytoma
            (2) Oligodendroglioma
            (3) Ependymoma
            (4) Meningioma
            (5) Pituitary adenoma
            (6) Craniopharyngioma
            (7) Pineal region tumor
            (8) Medulloblastoma
            (9) Hemangioblastoma
            (10) Chordoma
            (11) Primary CNS lymphoma
         b. Secondary
            (1) Lung
            (2) Breast
            (3) Melanoma
            (4) Colorectal

List Continues

DIFFERENTIAL DIAGNOSIS BY ETIOLOGY
(*Continued*)

    (5) Renal
    (6) Thyroid
    (7) Systemic lymphoma
  2. Cyst
    a. Dermoid cyst (mostly midline, also CP angle, parasellar, lumbosacral spine)
    b. Epidermoid cyst (CP angle, parasellar, LS spine)
    c. Mucocele (parasellar)
    d. Colloid cyst of third ventricle
    e. Arachnoid cyst
    f. Spinal epithelial cyst, enteric cyst
    g. Aneurysmal bone cyst (spinal)
  3. Granuloma (noninfectious)
    a. Tolosa-Hunt Syndrome/orbital pseudotumor
    b. Histiocytosis X
    c. Wegener's granulomatosis
    d. Lymphomatoid granulomatosis
B. Vascular malformation
  1. AVM
  2. Cavernous angioma
  3. Venous angioma
  4. Capillary hemangioma
C. Hematoma
  1. Hypertensive
  2. Aneurysm
  3. Subdural/epidural hematoma
  4. Secondary to vascular malformation
  5. Bleeding diathesis (leukemia, anticoagulants)
  6. Tumor (melanoma, renal cell, choriocarcinoma, hemangioblastoma)
  7. Amyloid angiopathy
D. Aneurysm
E. Congenital malformation
  1. Arnold-Chiari malformation
  2. Dandy-Walker deformity
  3. Basilar impression
F. Abscess/parasitic cyst
G. Hydrocephalus/syringomyelia/syringobulbia (e.g., normal pressure hydrocephalus)
H. Degenerative (e.g., herniated disc, spondylosis, and spinal stenosis)

DIFFERENTIAL DIAGNOSIS BY ETIOLOGY
(*Continued*)

III. Myelin (demyelinating/dysmyelinating, CNS or PNS)
    A. Multiple sclerosis
    B. Postinfectious demyelination
    C. Leukodystrophies (also under inherited disorders)
    D. Central pontine myelinolysis
    E. Marchiafava-Bignami syndrome
IV. Metabolic (other than inherited defect)
    A. Endocrine (diabetes, thyroid, parathyroid, adrenal, acromegaly)
    B. Drugs
    C. Toxins
    D. Nutritional (vitamins or other cofactors)
    E. Organ failure (e.g., uremia, electrolytes, hepatic failure, hypoxia)
V. Infectious (including skull/vertebrae, brain, cord, meninges, nerves, muscles)
    A. Bacterial
        1. Meningococcal influenza
        2. *Pneumococcus*
        3. *Listeria*
        4. TB
        5. Sarcoid
        6. *Staphylococcus*
        7. *Streptococcus* group A
        8. Coli, group B streptococcus in infants
        9. *Rickettsia*
      10. *Mycobacterium leprae*
    B. Viral
        1. RNA
            a. Enterovirus
                (1) Poliovirus
                (2) Echovirus
                (3) Coxsackievirus
            b. Arbovirus
            c. Influenza
            d. Measles
            e. Mumps
            f. Lymphocytic choriomeningitis
            g. Rabies

List Continues

DIFFERENTIAL DIAGNOSIS BY ETIOLOGY
(*Continued*)

2. DNA
   a. Herpesvirus
      (1) Simplex type I
      (2) Simplex type II in immunocompromised host
      (3) Varicella zoster
      (4) CMV
      (5) Epstein-Barr virus
   b. Adenovirus
3. "Slow virus"
   a. Progressive multifocal leukoencephalopathy
   b. Creutzfeldt-Jakob disease
   c. Subacute sclerosing panencephalitis
   d. Progressive rubella panencephalitis
   e. Kuru
4. HIV

C. Fungal
   1. *Cryptococcus*
   2. *Candida*
   3. Mucormycosis
   4. *Aspergillus*
   5. *Nocardia*
   6. Blastomycosis

D. Spirochetes
   1. Syphilis
   2. Lyme disease

E. Parasitic
   1. Helminths (worms)
      a. Trichinosis
      b. Schistosomiasis
      c. *Echinococcus* (hydatid cyst)
      d. Cysticercosis
   2. Protozoa (unicellular)
      a. Toxoplasmosis
      b. Trypanosomiasis
      c. Malaria
      d. Amebiasis

DIFFERENTIAL DIAGNOSIS BY ETIOLOGY
(*Continued*)

   VI. Neurodegenerative (of unknown etiology, other than inherited defect; e.g., Parkinson's or Alzheimer's disease)

  VII. Paraneoplastic (not mass lesions)
- A. Remote effects
- B. Meningeal carcinomatosis
- C. Paraproteins

VIII. Inherited neurometabolic disorder (includes inborn errors of metabolism, neurocutaneous syndromes, chromosomal defects, etc.)

   IX. Seizure (convulsive or nonconvulsive)

    X. Trauma
- A. Mechanical
- B. Radiation
- C. Thermal (hot or cold)
- D. Electrical

   XI. Psychogenic/psychiatric

INHERITED NEUROMETABOLIC DISORDERS

I. Carbohydrate
   A. Glycogenoses (see also Lysosomal storage)
      1. Acid maltase deficiency (type II, Pompe's disease)
      2. Debrancher enzyme deficiency (type III)
      3. Myophosphorylase deficiency (type V, McArdle's disease)
      4. Phosphofructokinase deficiency (type VII, Tarui's disease)
   B. Lafora body disease
   C. Galactosemia
II. Lipid and lipoprotein
   A. Alphalipoprotein deficiency (Tangier disease)
   B. Abetalipoproteinemia (Bassen-Kornzweig disease)
   C. Carnitine deficiency
   D. Carnitine palmityl transferase deficiency
III. Urea cycle (common feature is hyperammonemia)
   A. Type II hyperammonemia
   B. Citrullinemia
   C. Argininosuccinic aciduria
   D. Hyperornithinemia
IV. Amino/organic acid
   A. Phenylketonuria
   B. Maple syrup urine disease
   C. Homocystinuria
   D. Hartnup's disease
   E. Glutaric acidemia type I
   F. Methylmalonic aciduria
   G. Lesch-Nyhan syndrome
   H. Hyperalaninemia
V. Peroxisome
   A. Adrenoleukodystrophy
   B. Hereditary sensorimotor neuropathy type IV (Refsum's disease)
   C. Zellweger syndrome (cerebrohepatorenal syndrome)
VI. Mitochondrial encephalomyopathy
   A. MERRF (myoclonic epilepsy with red ragged fibers)
   B. MELAS (mitochondrial myopathy, encephalopathy, lactic acidosis, stroke-like episodes)
   C. Defects of the respiratory chain
      1. Complex I, III deficiency
      2. Complex IV (cytochrome c oxidase) deficiency
         a. Subacute necrotizing encephalomyelopathy (Leigh's disease)
         b. Fatal infantile mitochondrial myopathy

INHERITED NEUROMETABOLIC DISORDERS
(*Continued*)

    c. Benign infantile mitochondrial myopathy
    d. Trichopoliodystrophy (Menkes syndrome)
    e. Progressive sclerosing poliodystrophy (Alper syndrome)
VII. Lysosomal storage
  A. Lipidoses
    1. Cerebrotendinous xanthomatosis
    2. Fabry's disease
    3. Farber's disease
    4. Gaucher's disease
    5. GM_1 gangliosidosis
    6. GM_2 gangliosidosis (this heading includes a variety of early or later onset syndromes related to deficiency of one or more components of hexosaminidase complex [two alleles, alpha and beta, make possible three isoenzymes, A, B, and S])
    7. Krabbe's globoid body leukodystrophy
    8. Metachromatic leukodystrophy
    9. Neuronal ceroid-lipofuscinoses
      a. Infantile neuronal ceroid-lipofuscinosis (Santavuori-Haltia)
      b. Late infantile ceroid-lipofuscinosis (Jansky-Bielschowsky disease)
      c. Juvenile neuronal ceroid-lipofuscinosis (Spielmeyer-Vogt disease or Batten's disease)
      d. Adult neuronal ceroid lipofuscinosis (Kufs disease)
    10. Niemann-Pick disease
  B. Mucopolysaccharidoses
    1. Hurler syndrome
    2. Hunter syndrome
    3. Sanfilippo syndrome
    4. Morquio syndrome
    5. Maroteaux-Lamy syndrome
  C. Mucolipidoses
    1. Mannosidosis
    2. Fucosidosis
    3. Sialidoses
      a. Cherry-red spot myoclonus syndrome (type I)
      b. Type II
  D. Glycogenoses (see also Carbohydrate)
    1. Acid maltase deficiency (type II, Pompe's disease)
    2. Debrancher enzyme deficiency (type III)

List Continues

INHERITED NEUROMETABOLIC DISORDERS
(*Continued*)

      3. Myophosphorylase deficiency (type V, McArdle's disease)
      4. Phosphofructokinase deficiency (type VII, Tarui's disease)
VIII. Metal disorders
   A. Copper
      1. Wilson's disease
      2. Trichopoliodystrophy (Menkes disease)
   B. Iron
      1. Hallervorden-Spatz disease

PRACTICE GUIDELINES: NEUROLOGICAL EVALUATION

I. A physician who performs a neurological evaluation should be responsible for the following:
   A. Determining the neurological status of the patient
   B. Developing provisional and differential diagnose
   C. Developing a plan for further evaluation
   D. Communicating the proposed plan to the patient and family members
   E. Communicating the proposed plan to other pertinent physicians involved in the care of the patient
II. The development of an appropriate neurological diagnosis and care plan includes the following:
   A. Reviewing, or obtaining for later review, pertinent medical records
   B. Interviewing and examining the patient by
      1. Discussing the neurological history and defining the temporal evolution of the primary neurological symptoms and related neurological symptoms
      2. Assessing the relevant aspects of the findings on physical and neurological examination that relate to the neurological symptoms
   C. Defining the additional states and evaluations that may be needed to plan further care
   D. Defining the neurological care plan, including follow-up of results of diagnostic testing and therapy

This list of essential items should be part of the standard evaluation. It should help those in training develop a systematic approach to the neurological evaluation and improve the standard of care.

(From Report of the Quality Standards Subcommittee of the American Academy of Neurology: Practice guidelines: neurological evaluation. Neurology 40:871, 1990, with permission.)

PREVALENCE OF COMMON NEUROLOGICAL ENTITIES*

Disorder	Rate (per 100,000 population)
Migraine	2,000
Other forms of severe headaches	1,500
Brain injury	800
Epilepsy	6,500
Acute cerebrovascular disease	600
Lumbosacral pain syndrome (low back pain)	500
Alcoholism	500
Sleep disorders (narcolepsies and hypersomnias)	300
Ménière's disease	300
Lumbosacral herniated nucleus pulposus	300
Cerebral palsy	250
Dementia	250
Parkinsonism	200
Transient ischemic attacks	150
Febrile seizures	100
Persistent postconcussive syndrome	80
Herpes zoster	80
Congenital malformations of the CNS	70
Single seizures	60
Multiple sclerosis	60
Benign brain tumors	60
Cervical pain syndromes	60
Down syndrome	50
Subarachnoid hemorrhage	50
Cervical herniated nucleus pulposus	50
Spinal cord injury	50
Transient postconcussive syndrome	50

* Prevalence is the total number of cases of a disease existing at any one time. (From Kurtzke JF: The current neurological burden of illness in the United States. Neurology 32:1207–1214, 1982, with permission.)

PREVALENCE OF LESS COMMON NEUROLOGICAL ENTITIES

Disorder	Rate (per 100,000 population)
Tic douloureux	40
Neurological symptoms without a defined disease	40
Mononeuropathy	40
Polyneuropathy	40
Dorsolateral sclerosis	30
Peripheral nerve trauma	30
Other head injury	30
Hereditary atrophies/dystrophies	20
Metastatic brain tumor	15
Other demyelinating diseases	12
Chronic progressive myelopathy	10
Benign cord tumor	10
Encephalitides	10
Hereditary ataxias	8
Syrinx	7
Hereditary striatopallidal diseases	6
Motor neuron disease	6
Polymyositis	6
Malignant primary brain tumor	5
Metastatic cord tumor	5
Meningitides	5
Bell's palsy	5
Myasthenia gravis	4
Intracerebral abscess	2
Cranial nerve trauma	2
Guillain-Barré syndrome	1
Vascular disease of the spinal cord	1
Acute (transverse) myelopathy	1

(From Kurtzke JF: The current neurological burden of illness in the United States. Neurology 32:1207–1214, 1982, with permission.)

INCIDENCE OF COMMON NEUROLOGICAL ENTITIES*

Disorder	Rate (per 100,000 population)
Herpes zoster	400
Migraine	250
Brain trauma	200
Other forms of severe headache	200
Acute cerebrovascular disease	150
Other head injury	150
Transient postconcussive syndrome	150
Lumbosacral herniated nucleus pulposus	150
Lumbosacral pain syndrome (low back pain)	150
Neurological symptoms without a defined disease	75
Epilepsy	50
Febrile seizures	50
Dementia	50
Menière's disease	50
Mononeuropathies	40
Polyneuropathy	40
Transient ischemic attacks	30
Bell's palsy	25
Single seizures	20
Parkinsonism	20
Alcoholism	20
Persistent postconcussive syndrome	20
Cervical pain syndrome	20
Meningitides	15
Encephalitides	15
Sleep disorders	15
Subarachnoid hemorrhage	15
Cervical herniated nucleus pulposus	15
Metastatic brain tumor	15
Peripheral nerve trauma	15
Blindness	15
Benign brain tumor	10
Deafness	10

* Incidence is the number of new cases of a disorder beginning within the population during a period of time (usually 1 year).
(From Kurtzke JF: The current neurological burden of illness in the United States. Neurology 32:1207–1214, 1982, with permission.)

INCIDENCE OF LESS COMMON NEUROLOGICAL ENTITIES*

Disorder	Rate (per 100,000 population)
Cerebral palsy	9
Congenital malformations of the CNS	7
Mental retardation, other	6
Mental retardation, severe	6
Malignant primary brain tumor	5
Metastatic spinal cord tumor	5
Other demyelinating disease	4
Tic douloureux	4
Multiple sclerosis	3
Dorsolateral sclerosis	3
Functional psychosis	3
Spinal cord injury	3
Motor neuron disease	2
Down syndrome	2
Guillain-Barré syndrome	2
Hereditary atrophies/dystrophies	1.2
Intracranial abscess	1
Benign primary spinal cord tumor	1
Cranial nerve trauma	1
Hereditary striatopallidal disease	0.5
Chronic progressive myelopathy	0.5
Polymyositis	0.5
Syrinx	0.4
Hereditary ataxias	0.4
Myasthenia gravis	0.4
Acute (transverse) myelopathy	0.2
Malignant primary spinal cord tumor	0.1
Vascular disease of the spinal cord	0.1

* Incidence is the number of new cases of a disorder beginning within the population during a period of time (usually 1 year).
(From Kurtzke JF: The current neurological burden of illness in the United States. Neurology 32:1207–1214, 1982, with permission.)

CANADIAN NEUROLOGICAL SCALE*

Mentation	On Examination	Score
Level of consciousness	Alert	3
	Drowsy	1.5
Orientation	Oriented	1
	Disoriented or not applicable	0
Speech	Normal	1
	Expressive deficit	0.5
	Receptive deficit	0
Motor weakness		
Face	None	0.5
	Present	0
Arm: proximal	None	1.5
	Mild	1
	Significant	0.5
	Total	0
Arm: distal	None	1.5
	Mild	1
	Significant	0.5
	Total	0
Leg	None	1.5
	Mild	1
	Significant	0.5
	Total	0
If comprehension defect present, use motor response		
Face	Symmetrical	0.5
	Asymmetrical	0
Arms	Equal	1.5
	Unequal	0
Legs	Equal	1.5
	Unequal	0

* The Canadian Neurological Scale is in common use for patients with neurological diseases such as stroke or mild head trauma. It may be useful in monitoring patients and in the assessment of prognosis and therapy.

(From Coté R, Hachinski VC, Shurvell BL et al: The Canadian Neurological Scale: a preliminary study in acute stroke. Stroke 17:731–737, 1986, with permission.)

2
NEUROANATOMY/ NEURO- PHYSIOLOGY

COMMON FOCAL NEUROLOGICAL SIGNS AND THEIR ANATOMICAL LOCALIZATION

Syndrome	Localization
Hemiparesis, including facial weakness, hemisensory loss, aphasia, or hemianopia	Contralateral cerebral hemisphere
Hemiparesis without other findings	Usually small deep infarct (lacunar) in the contralateral cerebral hemisphere or pons
Hemiparesis with contralateral cranial nerve findings, often associated with cranial nerve signs	Brainstem
Bilateral pain and temperature loss with lower motor neuron signs at the level of the lesion (usually sparing lowest levels, "sacral sparing")	Central cord syndrome (e.g., syrinx)
Hemiparesis with contralateral loss of pain and temperature sense, and ipsilateral loss of vibration and position sense	Hemicord syndrome (Brown-Séquard syndrome)
Bilateral motor weakness and loss of pain and temperature sense, with preservation of vibration and position	Anterior cord syndrome
Bilateral loss of vibration and position sense	Posterior columns
Paraparesis	Thoracic or lower spinal cord or nerve roots (can also be seen with cerebral parasagittal lesions such as meningioma)
Monoparesis (most muscles of one arm or one leg)	Brachial or lumbar plexus lesion (need to exclude small lesion of cerebral cortex)

List Continues

COMMON FOCAL NEUROLOGICAL SIGNS AND THEIR ANATOMICAL LOCALIZATION (*Continued*)

Loss of pain and temperature sense in saddle distribution, marked sphincter and sexual dysfunction, mild motor findings in lower limbs (often symmetric); fasciculations may be present	Conus medullaris syndrome
Bilateral, often asymmetrical, motor and sensory (all modalities) deficits of lower lumbar (often more severe than with conus lesions) and sacral segments (sensory loss and pain in saddle distribution); bowel, bladder, and sexual dysfunction (late and mild)	Cauda equina syndrome
Weakness of isolated muscles of one limb	Peripheral nerve or spinal nerve root lesion
Bilateral distal limb numbness and/or weakness (legs usually worse)	Peripheral neuropathy
Bilateral proximal limb weakness without sensory symptoms	Muscle or neuromuscular junction (occasionally may be seen with neuropathies such as Guillain-Barré syndrome)

(Modified from Earnest MP: Principles of early diagnosis and management of nervous system emergencies. p. 1. In Neurologic Emergencies. Churchill Livingstone, New York, 1983, with permission.)

LIMBIC SYSTEM

PAPEZ' CIRCUIT

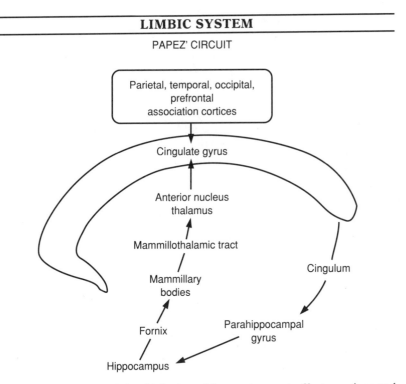

James Papez suggested that higher cognitive centers may affect emotions and visceral function; he proposed the pathway shown above, which now bears his name.

  I. Amygdala receives major afferents from olfactory system

 II. Amygdala has two major efferent projections

    A. Stria terminalis to bed nucleus of stria terminalis, septal area, nucleus accumbens, hypothalamus

    B. Ventral amygdalofugal pathway: hypothalamus, dorsomedial nucleus of thalamus, rostral cingulate gyrus

 III. Hippocampus receives major afferents from entorhinal cortex via the perforant pathway

 IV. Hippocampus has efferent projections via fornix to the following:

    A. Mammillary bodies

    B. Anterior intralaminar nucleus of thalamus

    C. Midbrain tegmentum

    D. Septal area, lateral preoptic area, hypothalamus

List Continues

LIMBIC SYSTEM (*Continued*)

V. Hypothalamus is divided into three groups of nuclei
   (Also receives input from retina to suprachiasmatic nucleus.)
   A. Periventricular
   B. Medial
   C. Lateral

(From Martin JH: Development as a guide to the regional anatomy of the brain. In Kandel ER, Schwartz JH (eds): Principles of Neural Science. Elsevier Science Publishing, New York, 1985, with permission.)

THALAMUS

I. Specific relay nuclei
   A. Anterior
      1. Function: limbic
      2. From mamillary bodies of hypothalamus
      3. To cingulate gyrus
   B. Ventral anterior (VA)
      1. Function: motor
      2. From globus pallidus
      3. To premotor cortex
   C. Ventral lateral (VL)
      1. Function: motor
      2. From dentate nucleus of cerebellum
      3. To motor premotor cortex
   D. Ventral posterior medial (face; VPM)
      1. Function: sensory
      2. From ascending sensory pathways
      3. To primary sensory cortex
   E. Ventral posterior lateral (body; VPL)
      1. Function: sensory
      2. From ascending sensory pathways
      3. To primary sensory cortex
   F. Medial geniculate
      1. Function: auditory
      2. From inferior colliculus via brachium of inferior colliculus
      3. To auditory cortex
   G. Lateral geniculate
      1. Function: visual
      2. From retinal ganglion cells
      3. To visual cortex
II. Association nuclei
   A. Lateral dorsal
      1. Function: emotional expression
      2. From cingulate gyrus
      3. To cingulate gyrus
   B. Lateral posterior
      1. Function: integration of sensory information
      2. From parietal lobe
      3. To parietal lobe

List Continues

THALAMUS (*Continued*)

  C. Pulvinar
    1. Function: integration of sensory information
    2. From superior colliculus; parietal, temporal, and occipital lobes; visual cortex
    3. To parietal, temporal, and occipital lobes
  D. Medial dorsal
    1. Function: limbic
    2. From amygdala, olfactory area, hypothalamus
    3. To prefrontal cortex
III. Nonspecific nuclei
  A. Midline nuclei
    1. Function: limbic
    2. From reticular formation, hypothalamus
    3. To basal forebrain
  B. Intralaminar nuclei
    1. From reticular formation, spinothalamic tract, globus pallidus, cortex
    2. To striatum (putamen)
  C. Reticular nucleus
    1. Function: modulation of thalamic activity
    2. From cortex, thalamic nuclei
    3. To thalamic nuclei

(Modified from Kelly JP: Anatomical basis of sensory perception and motor coordination. In Kandel ER, Schwartz JH (eds): Principles of Neural Science. Elsevier Science Publishing, New York, 1985, with permission.)

BASAL GANGLIA

MAJOR MOTOR CONTROL LOOPS OF THE BRAIN

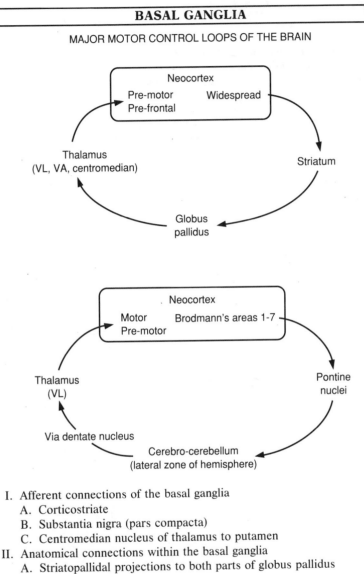

I. Afferent connections of the basal ganglia
   A. Corticostriate
   B. Substantia nigra (pars compacta)
   C. Centromedian nucleus of thalamus to putamen
II. Anatomical connections within the basal ganglia
   A. Striatopallidal projections to both parts of globus pallidus
   B. Striatonigral (pars reticulata)
   C. Intrastriatal interneurons
   D. Reciprocal innervation between globus pallidus and subthalamic nucleus

List Continues

BASAL GANGLIA (*Continued*)

III. Efferent projections from the basal ganglia
   A. Globus pallidus (internal) to thalamus (VA, VL, centromedian) via ansa lenticularis, lenticular fasciculus
   B. Substantia nigra, pars reticulata to thalamus (VA, VL)

(From Côté L, Crutcher MD: Motor functions of the basal ganglia and diseases of transmitter metabolism. In Kandel ER, Schwartz JH (eds): Principles of Neural Science. Elsevier Science Publishing, New York, 1985, with permission.)

CEREBELLUM

I. Three anatomical divisions
   A. The cerebellum can be divided into three lobes based on its *gross anatomical* appearance
      1. Anterior lobe
      2. Posterior lobe
      3. Flocculonodular lobe
II. Four divisions according to deep nuclear projections
   A. Different parts of the cerebellum project to different deep cerebellar nuclei; the cerebellum can thus be divided into four parts, in accordance with the *connections* to the four deep nuclei
      1. Flocculonodular lobe
         a. To vestibular nuclei
      2. Vermis: associated with ventromedial descending systems (proximal muscles)
         a. To fastigial nucleus
      3. Hemisphere (intermediate zone): associated with dorsolateral descending systems (distal muscles)
         a. To interposed nuclei (globose, emboliform)
      4. Hemisphere (lateral zone): associated with motor and premotor cortex
         a. To dentate nucleus
III. Three functional divisions
   A. Alternatively, the cerebellum can be classified into three distinct *functional* divisions
      1. Vestibulocerebellum (flocculonodular lobe): eye movements, equilibrium (axial muscles)
         a. From vestibular nuclei in medulla, semicircular canals (also from visual system)
         b. To vestibular nuclei in medulla, medial and lateral vestibulospinal tracts

List Continues

CEREBELLUM (*Continued*)

2. Spinocerebellum (vermis and intermediate zone of hemisphere): motor execution
   a. From spino/cuneocerebellar tracts (also from auditory, visual, vestibular systems; somatic sensory, motor cortex)
   b. Posterior spinocerebellar tract from Clarke's column is ipsilateral, enters via inferior cerebellar peduncle
   c. Anterior spinocerebellar tract from spinal border cells is bilateral, enters via superior cerebellar peduncle
   d. To fastigial nucleus (vermis, medial descending system, axial muscles)
   e. Reticular formation, lateral vestibular nucleus to spinal cord as reticulo/vestibulospinal tracts
   f. To contralateral motor cortex (axial part), then to spinal cord via anterior corticospinal tract
   g. To interposed nucleus (intermediate zone, lateral descending system, distal muscles)
   h. To contralateral red nucleus (magnocellular) via superior cerebellar peduncle, to contralateral spinal cord via rubrospinal tract
   i. To contralateral VL thalamus, to motor cortex (distal), to contralateral spinal cord via lateral corticospinal tract
3. Cerebrocerebellum (lateral zone of hemisphere): motor planning; no peripheral sensory input
   a. From pontine nuclei (via middle cerebellar peduncle), from contralateral cerebral cortex (motor, premotor, sensory, posterior parietal)
   b. To dentate nucleus to VL thalamus to motor, premotor cortex

CEREBELLUM (*Continued*)

IV. Cerebellar cortex
- A. The cerebellar cortex consists of three distinct layers, based on its *microscopic anatomy*
  - 1. Molecular cell layer
    - a. Parallel fibers (granule cell axons)
    - b. Inhibitory interneurons (basket, stellate) modulate Purkinje cells
  - 2. Purkinje cell layer
    - a. Dendrites up to molecular layer
    - b. Axons sole output of cerebellum (inhibitory)
  - 3. Granule cell layer
    - a. Granule cells project to molecular layer as parallel fibers
    - b. Golgi cells: inhibitory interneurons at glomeruli
    - c. Glomeruli (mossy fiber afferents)
- B. Two main cerebellar inputs (both synapse [excitatory] on deep nuclei on their way in)
  - 1. Mossy fibers
    - a. From brainstem nuclei, spinal cord
    - b. To glomeruli (granule cells) and Purkinje cells (via parallel fibers)
  - 2. Climbing fibers
    - a. From inferior olive
    - b. To Purkinje cells
  - 3. Also diffuse modulatory aminergic input
    - a. Serotonergic input from raphe nuclei
    - b. Noradrenergic input from locus ceruleus

(Modified from Ghez C, Fahn S: The cerebellum. In Kandel ER, Schwartz JH (eds): Principles of Neural Science. Elsevier Science Publishing, New York, 1985, with permission.)

CEREBELLAR PEDUNCLES

Peduncle	Afferents (In)	Efferents (Out)
Superior cerebellar	Ventral spinocerebellar (tectocerebellar; trigeminocerebellar)	Dentothalamic Globose → red nucleus Emboliform → inferior olive → reticular formation
Middle cerebellar	Corticopontocerebellar	None
Inferior cerebellar (restiform body)	Dorsal spinocerebellar, direct vestibulocerebellar, olivocerebellar, accessory inferior olivocerebellar	Fastigiobulbar (especially lateral vestibular nucleus), flocculonodular → vestibular

SKULL FORAMINA

Foramen	Structures Passing Through
Optic	Optic nerve Ophthalmic artery
Superior orbital fissure	Oculomotor nerve Trochlear nerve Abducens nerve Trigeminal nerve (ophthalmic division, V_1)
Foramen rotundum	Trigeminal nerve (maxillary division, V_2)
Foramen ovale	Trigeminal nerve (mandibular division, V_3) Lesser petrosal nerve
Foramen spinosum	Middle meningeal artery Meningeal branch of mandibular nerve
Foramen lacerum	Carotid artery enters into side above closed inferior portion
Carotid canal	Carotid artery Sympathetic plexus
Stylomastoid	Facial nerve (exit)
Internal acoustic meatus	Facial nerve Acoustic and vestibular nerves Labyrinthine artery and vein
Jugular foramen	Glossopharyngeal nerve Vagus nerve Accessory nerve Sigmoid sinus Inferior petrosal sinus
Foramen magnum	Spinal cord Hypoglossal nerve Vertebral arteries Spinal (anterior and posterior) arteries Cervical components of accessory nerve

MAJOR SPINAL CORD TRACTS

Tract	Origin	Termination	Function	Clinical Syndrome
Corticospinal	Contralateral cerebral cortex	Ventral horn	The major motor pathway	Ipsilateral upper motor neuron syndrome with weakness, spasticity, increased reflexes, and B abinski response
Lateral spinothalamic	Contralateral dorsal horn	Thalamus (VPL) and reticular formation	One of two major sensory (ascending) pathways—carries pain and temperature as well as crude touch	Contralateral loss of pain and temperature 1–3 segments below the site of the lesion
Dorsal columns	Skin, joint receptors, muscle spindles, Golgi tendon organs (cell bodies in dorsal root ganglia)	Nucleus gracilis (for leg) and nucleus cuneatus (for arm)	Second major sensory pathway—carries vibration, joint position sense, and fine touch	Ipsilateral loss of vibration and joint position sense, and fine discrimination for touch
Anterior (ventral) spinocerebellar	Joints, tendons, and muscle spindles via spinal border cells	Cerebellum (via superior cerebellar peduncle)	An afferent pathway for coordination of motor activity	Isolated syndrome not seen; usually involved in degenerative ataxic diseases (e.g., Friedreich's ataxia)
Posterior (dorsal) spinocerebellar	Joints, tendons, and muscle spindles via Clarke's column	Cerebellum (via inferior cerebellar peduncle)	An afferent pathway for coordination of motor activity	Isolated syndrome not seen; usually involved in degenerative ataxic diseases (e.g., Friedreich's ataxia)

BRACHIAL PLEXUS

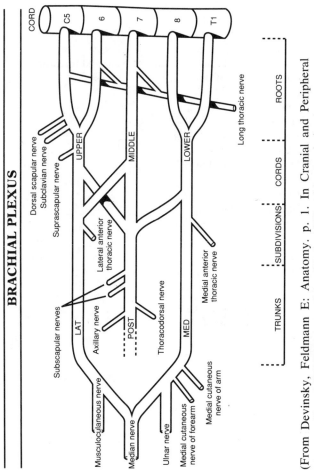

(From Devinsky, Feldmann E: Anatomy. p. 1. In Cranial and Peripheral Nerves. Churchill Livingstone, New York, 1988, with permission.)

DERMATOMAL DISTRIBUTION OF PAIN

CNV	Anterior cranium and facial structures
C2	Back of the Head
C3	Neck
C4	Epaulet
C5	Over deltoid muscle
C6	Radial forearm and thumb
C7	Index and middle finger
C8	Little finger and ulnar surface of hand and forearm
T1	Medial aspect of upper arm
T4–T5	Nipples
T10	Umbilicus
L1	Groin
L2	Anterior and lateral thigh
L3	Medial side of knee
L4	Medial aspect of lower leg
L5	Great toe
S1	Little toe
S2	Back of the thigh
S3–S5	Genitoanal

SOMATOSENSORY RECEPTORS

Receptor Type	Probable Function
Free nerve ending	Pain, temperature, touch
Hair follicle ending	Touch
Krause's end bulb	Touch, cold
Meissner's corpuscle	Touch, pressure (fine touch—lips and fingertips)
Merkel's disc	Touch, pressure (fine touch including areas with hair)
Pacinian corpuscle	Touch, pressure, vibration
Ruffini's corpuscle	Touch, warmth

TABLE OF AUTONOMIC INNERVATION

	Preganglionic Neuron	Postganglionic Neuron	Function
Head			
Eye: pupillary and ciliary muscles			
Sympathetic	Cord segments T1–T2	Superior cervical ganglion	Mydriasis, accommodation for far vision
Parasympathetic	Edinger-Westphal nucleus (CN III)	Ciliary ganglion	Miosis, accommodation for near vision
Lacrimal gland			
Sympathetic	Cord segments T1–T2	Superior cervical ganglion	Vasoconstriction
Parasympathetic	Lacrimal part of superior salivatory nucleus (CN VII)	Sphenopalatine ganglion	Tear secretion and vasodilation
Salivary glands			
Sympathetic	Upper thoracic cord segments	Superior cervical ganglion	Salivary secretion (mucous—low enzyme)
Parasympathetic parotid	Inferior salivatory nucleus (CN IX)	Otic ganglion	Salivary secretion (watery—high enzyme)
Submandibular/ sublingual	Superior salivatory nucleus (CN VII)	Submandibular ganglion	Salivary secretion (watery—high enzyme)
Thoracic viscera			
Heart			
Sympathetic	Cord segments T1–T4	Upper thoracic to superior cervical chain ganglia	Increase in heart rate and force of contraction; coronary vasodilation

Parasympathetic	Dorsal motor nucleus of vagus (CN X)	Cardiac plexus	Decrease in heart rate and force of contraction; coronary vasoconstriction
Esophagus			
Sympathetic	Thoracic cord segments	Thoracic and cervical chain ganglia	Vasoconstriction
Parasympathetic	Dorsal motor nucleus of vagus (CN X)	Intramural plexuses	Peristalsis and secretion
Lungs			
Sympathetic	Cord segments T2–T6	Thoracic chain ganglia	Bronchial dilation
Parasympathetic	Dorsal motor nucleus of vagus (CN X)	Pulmonary plexus	Bronchial constriction
Abdominal viscera			
Stomach and intestine			
Sympathetic	Cord segments T5–T12 (thoracic splanchnic nerves)	Celiac and superior mesenteric ganglia	Inhibition of peristalsis and secretion; sphincter contraction
Parasympathetic	Dorsal motor nucleus of vagus (CN X)	Intramural plexuses	Peristalsis and secretion
Adrenal medulla			
Sympathetic	Cord segments T8–T11 (thoracic splanchnic nerves)	Adrenomedullary cells are derived from neural crests but have no dendrites or axons—they are endocrine cells	Secretion of epinephrine
Parasympathetic	None		

List Continues

TABLE OF AUTONOMIC INNERVATION (*Continued*)

Head	Preganglionic Neuron	Postganglionic Neuron	Function
Descending colon			
Sympathetic	Cord segments T12–L2 (lumbar splanchnic nerves)	Inferior mesenteric ganglion	Inhibition of peristalsis and secretion; vasoconstriction
Parasympathetic	Cord segments S2–S4 (pelvic splanchnic nerves)	Intramural plexuses	Peristalsis and secretion
Pelvic viscera Sigmoid colon, rectum, anus, bladder, gonads and associated ducts and organs, and erectile tissue			
Sympathetic	Cord segments T12–L2 (lumbar splanchnic nerves)	Inferior mesenteric ganglion (hypogastric nerves)	Inhibition of peristalsis and secretion; anal and bladder sphincter contraction; vasoconstriction; ejaculation
Parasympathetic	Cord segments S2–S4 (pelvic splanchnic nerves)	Intramural or organ plexuses	Peristalsis and secretion; bladder detrusor muscle contraction; penile and clitoral erection

(From Bird TD: Autonomic nervous system dysfunction. p. 304. In Swanson PD: Signs & Symptoms in Neurology. JB Lippincott, Philadelphia, 1984, with permission.)

Neurotransmitters

ACETYLCHOLINE

I. Synthetic pathways

$$\text{Acetyl-CoA} + \text{choline}$$
$$\downarrow \quad \text{choline acetyl transferase}$$
$$\text{(CAT)}$$
$$\text{acetylcholine} + \text{CoA}$$

II. Cholinergic neurons
   A. Cortical Betz cells
   B. Motor neurons (peripheral nicotinic NMJ receptors on skeletal muscle)
   C. Motor neurons on Renshaw cells (central nicotinic receptors)
   D. Medial septal nuclei
   E. Diagonal band of Broca
   F. Nucleus basalis of Meynert
   G. All preganglionic autonomic neurons (nicotinic receptors on postganglionic neurons, distinct from neuromuscular junction)
   H. Parasympathetic postganglionic autonomic neurons
   I. Intrastriatal interneurons

BIOGENIC AMINES

I. Catecholamines
   A. Synthetic pathways

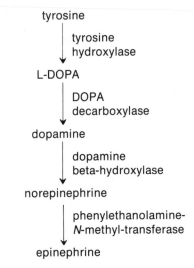

   B. Dopaminergic neurons
     1. Interplexiform cells innervating retinal horizontal cells
     2. Nigro striatal (pars compacta) system
     3. Mesolimbic: ventral tegmental area projects to limbic system (nucleus accumbens, olfactory tubercle, amygdala, frontal neocortex)
     4. Tuberoinfundibular: arcuate nucleus of median eminence to pituitary stalk
   C. Norepinephrine
     1. May be excitatory (alpha 1) by decreasing potassium conductance or inhibitory (alpha 2) by increasing potassium conductance
     2. Acts slowly via cAMP
       a. Noradrenergic neurons
       b. Locus ceruleus to cerebellum, neocortex
       c. Postganglionic sympathetic
       d. Lateral tegmentum of reticular formation

BIOGENIC AMINES (*Continued*)

II. Serotonin
  A. Synthetic pathways

tryptophan

    │ tryptophan
    ↓ hydroxylase

5-hydroxytryptophan

    │ 5-hydroxytryptophan
    ↓ decarboxylase

serotonin
(5-hydroxytryptamine)

  B. Serotonergic neurons
    1. Median raphe nuclei (usually generate IPSP by increased potassium conductance)

III. Histamine
  A. Synthetic pathways

histidine

    │ histidine
    ↓ decarboxylase

histamine

  B. Histaminergic neurons
    1. Hypothalamus

AMINO ACIDS

I. Aspartate-releasing neurons
   A. Neocortical pyramidal cells
   B. Primary sensory afferents
   C. Excitatory spinal cord interneurons
II. Glutamate-releasing neurons
   A. Primary sensory afferents
   B. Excitatory spinal cord interneurons
   C. Retinal receptors (rods, cones, excitatory or inhibitory, determined by type of bipolar cell)
   D. Hippocampus
   E. Neocortical pyramidal cells
III. Gamma-aminobutiric acid (GABA; inhibitory)
   A. Synthetic pathways

$$\text{glutamate}$$
$$\downarrow \quad \text{glutamic acid decarboxylase}$$
$$\text{GABA}$$
$$\downarrow \quad \text{GABA-transaminase (GABA-T)}$$
$$\text{succinic semialdehyde}$$

   B. GABA-ergic neurons
     1. Spinal cord inhibitory interneurons: presynaptic inhibition (also postsynaptic)
       a. GABA-A receptors on primary afferent terminals
     2. Olfactory granule cells
     3. Amacrine cells of the retina
     4. Purkinje cells
     5. Basket cells in cerebellum and hippocampus
     6. Striatonigral projection
     7. Striatopallidal projection
     8. Neocortical basket cells (interneurons)
IV. Glycine-releasing neurons (inhibitory)
   A. Spinal cord inhibitory interneurons (reciprocal inhibition)
   B. Spinal cord inhibitory interneurons: Renshaw cells (recurrent inhibition)

3
NEUROLOGICAL EXAMINATION

MENTAL STATUS EXAM

I. Level of consciousness, orientation
II. Attention
    A. Serial sevens
    B. Repetition of digits forward and backward
    C. Recite days of week, months of year, letters of alphabet, forward or backward
III. Language
    A. Spontaneous speech
    B. Comprehension
    C. Repetition
    D. Naming
    E. Reading
    F. Writing
IV. Memory
    A. Immediate
    B. Recent
    C. Remote
V. Visual-spatial
    A. Draw a clock reading "10 after 11"
    B. Copy figures
    C. Draw a cube
VI. Proverbs
VII. Praxis
    A. Ideomotor
    B. Ideational
VIII. Others
    A. Judgment
    B. Insight
    C. Affect

CRANIAL NERVES

Cranial Nerve	Origin	Function	Course of the Nerve
I. Olfactory (sensory)	Bipolar olfactory neurons	Smell	Central axons of bipolar neurons pass through cribriform plate of ethmoid bone and synapse in olfactory bulb.
II. Optic (sensory)	Retinal ganglion cells	Vision	Axons of ganglion cells converge at optic disc to form optic nerve, which passes through optic foramen.
III. Oculomotor Parasympathetic	Edinger-Westphal nucleus (upper midbrain)	Sphincter muscle of iris, ciliary muscle	Exits ventral midbrain near midline; runs parallel to posterior communicating artery, then traverses cavernous sinus and enters orbit through the superior orbital fissure.
Motor	Oculomotor nucleus (upper midbrain)	Superior, inferior, and medial rectus muscles; inferior oblique muscle; levator palpabrae superioris muscle	
IV. Trochlear (motor)	Trochlear nucleus (lower midbrain)	Superior oblique muscle	Fibers from the nucleus cross in anterior medullary velum and exit dorsally, below the colliculi; nerve traverses cavernous sinus

| | | | after winding around midbrain; enters orbit through superior orbital fissure. |

Nerve	Nucleus/Ganglion	Function	Course
V. Trigeminal			
Motor	Motor nucleus of CN V (pons)	Muscles of mastication	Ophthalmic division (V_1) passes through superior orbital fissure.
Sensory (somatic)	Semilunar (trigeminal) ganglion	Tactile sensation to skin of face, mucosa of nose and mouth, and dura	Maxillary division (V_2) passes through foramen rotundum; mandibular division (V_3) passes through foramen ovale.
VI. Abducens (motor)	Abducens nucleus (pons)	Lateral rectus muscle	Exits ventral pons near midline, ascends and curves around petrous tip; traverses cavernous sinus and enters orbit through superior orbital fissure; long course.
VII. Facial			
Parasympathetic	Superior salivatory nucleus (pons)	Lacrimal gland and mucous membranes of mouth and nose; submandibular and sublingual salivery glands	Exits lower pons laterally and passes through internal auditory meatus into middle ear (where chorda tympani branch arises to carry taste fibers), then enters facial canal and exits cranium through stylomastoid foramen; divides into terminal branches in the parotid gland.

List Continues

CRANIAL NERVES (Continued)

Cranial Nerve	Origin	Function	Course of the Nerve
Motor	Main motor nucleus (pons)	Muscles of facial expression	
Sensory (somatic)	Geniculate ganglion	Tactile sensation to parts of external ear, auditory canal, and external tympanic membrane.	
Sensory (special)	Geniculate ganglion	Taste sensation to the anterior two-thirds of tongue	
VIII. Vestibulocochlear			Vestibular and cochlear nerves join in the internal auditory meatus and enter the brainstem at the cerebellopontine angle.
Vestibular nerve (special sensory)	Vestibular ganglion	Equilibrium (supplies semicircular canals, utricle, and saccule)	
Cochlear nerve (special sensory)	Spiral ganglion	Hearing (supplies organ of Corti)	
IX. Glossopharyngeal			Attaches to the rostral medulla near the posterolateral sulcus; exits cranium through jugular foramen.
Parasympathetic	Inferior salivatory nucleus (medulla)	Supplies parotid gland	
Motor	Nucleus ambiguus (medulla)	Stylopharyngeus muscle	
Sensory (somatic)	Superior ganglion	Tactile sensation to posterior third of tongue, pharynx, middle ear, eustachian tube, and dura	
Sensory (special)	Inferior ganglion	Taste sensation to the posterior third of tongue	

X. Vagus			
Parasympathetic	Dorsal motor nucleus of CN X (medulla)	Viscera of thorax and abdomen	Attaches to mid-medulla near the posterolateral sulcus; exits cranium through jugular foramen.
Motor	Nucleus ambiguus (medulla)	Muscles of pharynx and larynx	
Sensory (somatic)	Superior ganglion	Tactile sensation to dura and auditory canal	
Sensory (visceral afferents)	Inferior ganglion	Viscera of thorax and abdomen	
XI. Accessory			
Motor—cranial	Nucleus ambiguus (medulla)	Muscles of larynx	Cranial fibers pass in CN XI, then join CN X, and then in the recurrent laryngeal nerve; spinal fibers ascend and enter cranium through the foramen magnum, then join the cranial fibers (in CN X) and exit the cranium through jugular foramen, and then separate from cranial fibers.
Motor—spinal	Anterior gray horn of cervical cord	Sternocleidomastoid and trapezius muscles	
XII. Hypoglossal (motor)	Hypoglossal nucleus (lower medulla)	Intrinsic muscles of tongue; genioglossus, hyoglossus, and styloglossus muscles	Attaches to the lower medulla near the anterolateral sulcus; exits cranium through the hypoglossal canal (occipital bone).

(From Devinsky O, Feldmann E: Anatomy. Examination of the Cranial and Peripheral Nerves. Churchill Livingstone, New York, 1988, with permission.)

SEGMENTAL AND PERIPHERAL INNERVATION TO THE MUSCLES AND THEIR FUNCTION

Nerve/Muscle	Function	Spinal Segments
Spinal accessory		
Trapezius	Elevates shoulder/arm	
	Fixes scapula	C3C4
Phrenic diaphragm	Inspiration	C3C4C5
Dorsal scapular		
Rhomboids	Draw scapula up and in	C4C5C6
Levator scapulae	Elevates scapula	C3C4C5
Long thoracic		
Serratus anterior	Fixes scapula on arm raise	C5C6C7
Anterior thoracic		
Pectoralis major (clavicular)	Pulls shoulder forward	C5C6
Pectoralis major (sternal)	Adducts and medially rotates arm	C6C7C8T1
Pectoralis minor	Depresses scapula, pulls shoulder forward	C6C7C8
Suprascapular		
Supraspinatus	Abducts humerus	C5C6
Infraspinatus	Rotates humerus laterally	C5C6
Subscapular		
Subscapularis	Rotates humerus medially	C5C6
Teres major	Adducts, medially rotates humerus	C5C6C7
Thoracodorsal		
Latissimus dorsi	Adducts, medially rotates humerus	C6C7C8
Axillary		
Teres minor	Adducts, laterally rotates humerus	C5C6
Deltoid	Abducts arm	C5C6

Nerve / Muscle	Action	Level
Musculocutaneous		
Coracobrachialis	Flexes and adducts arm	C6**C7**
Biceps brachii	Flexes and supinates arm	**C5**C6
Brachialis	Flexes forearm	**C5**C6
Radial		
Triceps	Extends forearm	C6**C7**C8
Brachioradialis	Flexes forearm	**C5**C6
Extensor carpi radialis (longus and brevis)	Extend wrist, abduct hand	**C5**C6
Posterior interosseus		
Supinator	Supinates forearm	C6**C7**
Extensor carpi ulnaris	Extends wrist, adducts hand	**C7**C8
Extensor digitorum	Extends fingers at proximal phalanx	**C7**C8
Extensor digiti quinti	Extends little finger at proximal phalanx	**C7**C8
Abductor pollicis longus	Abducts thumb in the plane of palm	**C7**C8
Extensor pollicis (longus and brevis)	Extend thumb	**C7**C8
Extensor indicis	Extends index finger, proximal phalanx	**C7**C8
Median		
Pronator teres	Pronates and flexes forearm	C6**C7**
Flexor carpi radialis	Flexes wrist, abducts hand	C6**C7**
Palmaris longus	Flexes wrist	**C7C8**T1
Flexor digitorum superficialis	Flexes middle phalanges	**C7C8**T1
Flexor digitorum profundus (digits 2 and 3)	Flexes distal phalanges	**C7C8**
Abductor pollicis brevis	Abducts thumb at right angles to palm	**C8T1**
Flexor pollicis brevis (superficial)	Flexes first phalanx of thumb	**C8T1**
Opponenes pollicis	Flexes, opposes thumb	**C8T1**
Lumbricals (I and II)	Flex proximal interphalangeal joint, extend other phalanges	**C8T1**
Anterior interosseus		
Flexor digitorum profundus (digits 2 and 3)	Flexes distal phalanges	**C7C8**
Flexor pollicis longus	Flexes distal phalanx of thumb	**C7C8**
Pronator quadratus	Pronates forearm	**C7C8**T1

List Continues

SEGMENTAL AND PERIPHERAL INNERVATION TO THE MUSCLES
AND THEIR FUNCTION (Continued)

Nerve/Muscle	Function	Spinal Segments
Ulnar		
Flexor carpi ulnaris	Flexes wrist, adducts hand	C7**C8**T1
Flexor digitorum profundus (digits 4 and 5)	Flexes distal phalanges	C7**C8**
Hypothenar muscles	Abduct, adduct, flex, rotate digit 5	**C8T1**
Lumbricals (III and IV)	Flex proximal interphalangeal joint, extend other phalanges	**C8T1**
Palmar interossei	Adduct fingers, flex proximal phalanges	**C8T1**
Dorsal interrossei	Adduct fingers	**C8T1**
Flexor pollicis brevis (deep)	Flexes and adducts thumb	**C8T1**
Adductor pollicis	Adducts thumb	**C8T1**
Obturator		
Obturator externus	Adducts and outwardly rotates leg	**L2**L3L4
Adductor longus		
Adductor magnus	Adduct thigh	**L2**L3L4
Adductor brevis		
Gracilis		
Femoral		
Iliacus	Flexes leg at hip	L1**L2**L3
Rectus femoris		
Vastus lateralis		
Vastus intermedius	Extend leg	**L2**L3L4
Vastus medialis		
Pectineus	Adducts leg	**L2**L3L4
Sartorius	Inwardly rotates leg, flexes thigh and leg	**L2**L3L4
Sciatic		
Adductor magnus	Adducts thigh	L4**L5**S1
Semitendinosus	Flexes and medially rotates knee, extends hip	**L5S1**S2

Muscle	Action	Innervation
Biceps femoris	Flexes leg, extends thigh	**L5S1S2**
Semimembranosus	Flexes and medially rotates knee, extends hip	**L5S1S2**
Tibial		
Gastrocnemius	Plantar flexes foot	S1S2
Plantaris	Spreads, brings together, and flexes proximal phalanges	L4L5S1
Soleus	Plantar flexes foot	S1S2
Popliteus	Plantar flexes foot	L4L5S1
Tibialis posterior	Plantar flexes and inverts foot	L4L5
Flexor digitorum longus	Flexes distal phalanges, aids plantar flexion	L5**S1S2**
Flexor hallucis longus	Flexes great toe, aids plantar flexion	L5**S1S2**
Small foot muscles	Cup sole	S1S2
Common peroneal		
Superficial peroneal		
Peroneus longus	Plantar flexes and everts foot	L5S1
Peroneus brevis	Plantar flexes and everts foot	L5S1
Deep peroneal		
Tibialis anterior	Dorsiflexes and inverts foot	**L4L5**
Extensor digitorum longus	Extends phalanges, dorsiflexes foot	**L5S1**
Extensor hallucis longus	Extends great toe, aids dorsiflexion	**L5S1**
Peroneus tertius	Plantar flexes foot in pronation	L4**L5S1**
Extensor digitorum brevis	Extends toes	L5S1
Superior gluteal		
Gluteus medius/minimus	Abduct and medially rotate thigh	**L4L5S1**
Tensor fasciae latae	Flexes thigh	**L4L5S1**
Inferior gluteal		
Gluteus maximus	Extends, abducts, laterally rotates thigh and extends lower trunk	**L5S1S2**

* Muscles are listed in the order of innervation, except when presented in groups, as for the quadriceps. Boldface type signifies predominant innervation.
(From Devinsky O, Feldmann E: Anatomy. p. 1. In Examination of the Cranial and Peripheral Nerves. Churchill Livingstone, New York, 1988, with permission.)

MUSCLES ACTING ON THE JOINTS

I. Muscles acting on the temporomandibular joint
  A. Open mouth
    1. Lateral pterygoid
    2. Digastric
    3. Geniohyoid
    4. Mylohyoid
  B. Close mouth
    1. Masseter
    2. Temporalis
    3. Medial pterygoid
  C. Protrude jaw
    1. Lateral pterygoid
    2. Medial pterygoid
  D. Laterally displace jaw toward opposite side
    1. Lateral pterygoid
    2. Medial pterygoid
II. Muscles acting on the shoulder girdle and joint
  A. Elevation
    1. Trapezius (upper fibers)
    2. Sternocleidomastoid
    3. Levator scapulae
    4. Rhomboids—major and minor
  B. Forward displacement (protraction)
    1. Pectoralis minor
    2. Serratus anterior
  C. Backward displacement (retraction)
    1. Trapezius
    2. Rhomboids—major and minor
  D. Flexion
    1. Pectoralis major (clavicular fibers)
    2. Coracobrachialis
    3. Deltoid (anterior fibers)
    4. Biceps
  E. Extension
    1. Deltoid (posterior fibers)
    2. Triceps
    3. Teres major
    4. Latissimus dorsi
  F. Adduction
    1. Pectoralis major
    2. Triceps

MUSCLES ACTING ON THE JOINTS (*Continued*)

      3. Teres major
      4. Latissimus dorsi
      5. Subscapularis
   G. Abduction
      1. Deltoid
      2. Supraspinatus
   H. Internal (medial) rotation
      1. Pectoralis major
      2. Deltoid (anterior fibers)
      3. Teres major
      4. Latissimus dorsi
      5. Subscapularis
    I. External (lateral) rotation
      1. Deltoid (posterior fibers)
      2. Infraspinatus
      3. Teres minor

III. Muscles acting on the elbow joint
   A. Extension
      1. Triceps
      2. Anconeus
      3. Extensor carpi radialis longus
      4. Extensor carpi radialis brevis
      5. Extensor carpi ulnaris
      6. Extensor digitorum
      7. Supinator
   B. Flexion
      1. Biceps
      2. Brachialis
      3. Brachioradialis
      4. Flexor carpi radialis
      5. Flexor carpi ulnaris
      6. Pronator teres
      7. Flexor digitorum superficialis
      8. Palmaris longus
   C. Supination
      1. Biceps
      2. Supinator
      3. Extensor pollicis longus
   D. Pronation
      1. Pronator teres
      2. Pronator quadratus

List Continues

MUSCLES ACTING ON THE JOINTS (*Continued*)

IV. Muscles acting on the wrist joint
   A. Flexion
      1. Flexor carpi ulnaris
      2. Flexor carpi radialis
      3. Palmaris longus
      4. Flexor digitorum profundus
      5. Flexor digitorum superficialis
      6. Flexor pollicis longus
   B. Extension
      1. Extensor carpi ulnaris
      2. Extensor carpi radialis longus
      3. Extensor carpi radialis brevis
      4. Extensor digitorum
      5. Extensor pollicis longus
      6. Extensor indicis
      7. Extensor digiti minimi
   C. Adduction
      1. Flexor carpi ulnaris
      2. Extensor carpi ulnaris
   D. Abduction
      1. Extensor carpi radialis longus
      2. Extensor carpi radialis brevis
      3. Flexor carpi radialis
      4. Extensor pollicis longus
      5. Extensor pollicis brevis
      6. Abductor pollicis longus
V. Muscles acting at the finger joints (digits 2–5)
   A. Flexion
      1. Flexor digitorum profundus (distal phalanges; digits 2–5)
      2. Flexor digitorum superficialis (middle and proximal phalanges; digits 2–5)
      3. Palmar interossei (proximal phalanges; digits 2, 4, 5)
      4. Dorsal introssei (proximal phalanges; digits 2–5)
   B. Extension
      1. Extensor digitorum (all phalanges; digits 2–5)
      2. Extensor digiti minimi (all phalanges; digit 5)
      3. Extensor indicis (all phalanges; digit 2)
      4. Palmar interossei (distal phalanges; digits 2, 4, 5)
      5. Dorsal interossei (distal phalanges; digits 2–5)
   C. Adduction
      1. Palmar interossei (digits 2, 4, 5)

MUSCLES ACTING ON THE JOINTS (*Continued*)

   D. Abduction
   1. Dorsal interossei (digits 2, 4, 5)
   2. Extensor digitorum (digits 2, 4, 5)
   3. Extensor digiti minimi (digit 5)
   4. Abductor digiti minimi (digit 5)
   5. Extensor indicis (digit 2)
   E. Opposition
   1. Opponens digiti minimi (digit 5; draws metacarpal forward and rotates it medially)
VI. Muscle acting at the thumb joints
   A. Flexion
   1. Flexor pollicis longus (both phalanges)
   2. Flexor pollicis brevis (proximal phalanx and metacarpal)
   3. Opponens pollicis (metacarpal)
   B. Extension
   1. Extensor pollicis longus (both phalanges and metacarpal)
   2. Extensor pollicis brevis (proximal phalanx and metacarpal)
   3. Abductor pollicis longus (proximal phalanx and metacarpal)
   C. Adduction
   1. Adductor pollicis (proximal phalanx)
   D. Abduction
   1. Abductor pollicis longus (metacarpal)
   2. Abduuctor pollicis brevis (proximal phalanx and metacarpal)
   E. Opposition
   1. Opponens pollicis (flexes metacarpal and draws it medially)
VII. Muscles acting on the hip joint
   A. Flexion
   1. Iliacus
   2. Rectus femoris
   3. Pectineus
   4. Sartorius
   5. Tensor fasciae latae
   6. Adductors
   B. Extension
   1. Gluteus maximus
   2. Biceps femoris
   3. Semimembranosus
   4. Semitendinosus
   5. Adductor magnus
   C. Adduction
   1. Adductor magnus

List Continues

MUSCLES ACTING ON THE JOINTS (*Continued*)

    2. Adductor longus
    3. Adductor brevis
    4. Pectineus
    5. Gracilis
    6. Quadratus femoris
    7. Obturator externus
  D. Abduction
    1. Gluteus medius
    2. Gluteus minimus
    3. Tensor fasciae latae
    4. Piriformis
    5. Sartorius
  E. Medial (internal) rotation
    1. Gluteus medius
    2. Gluteus minimus
    3. Tensor fasciae latae
  F. Lateral (external) rotation
    1. Obturator internus
    2. Obturator externus
    3. Piriformis
    4. Gluteus maximus
    5. Adductors
    6. Gemelli
    7. Quadratus femoris
VIII. Muscles acting on the knee joint
  A. Flexion
    1. Biceps femoris
    2. Semimembranosus
    3. Semitendinosus
    4. Gracilis
    5. Sartorius
    6. Gastrocnemius
    7. Popliteus
    8. Plantaris
  B. Extension
    1. Quadricips femoris
    2. Tensor fasciae latae
  C. Medial (internal) rotation
    1. Semimembranosus
    2. Semitendinosus
    3. Popliteus

MUSCLES ACTING ON THE JOINTS (*Continued*)

      4. Gracilis
      5. Sartorius
    D. Lateral (external) rotation
      1. Biceps femoris
 IX. Muscles acting on the ankle joint
    A. Dorsiflexion
      1. Tibialis anterior
      2. Extensor digitorum longus
      3. Extensor hallucis longus
      4. Peroneus tertius
    B. Plantar flexion
      1. Soleus
      2. Gastrocnemius
      3. Tibialis posterior
      4. Flexor hallucis longus
      5. Plantaris
      6. Peroneus longus
      7. Peroneus brevis
    C. Inversion
      1. Tibialis anterior
      2. Tibialis posterior
      3. Flexor digitorum (medial fibers)
      4. Flexor hallucis longus
    D. Eversion
      1. Peroneus longus
      2. Peroneus brevis
      3. Extensor digitorum longus (lateral fibers)
      4. Peroneus tertius
  X. Muscles acting on the toes
    A. Flexion
      1. Flexor digitorum longus
      2. Flexor digitorum brevis
      3. Flexor hallucis longus
      4. Abductor hallucis
      5. Adductor hallucis
      6. Abductor digiti minimi
      7. Interossei (proximal phalanx)
    B. Extension
      1. Extensor digitorum longus
      2. Extensor digitorum brevis
      3. Extensor hallucis longus

List Continues

MUSCLES ACTING ON THE JOINTS (*Continued*)

4. Lumbricals
5. Interossei (distal phalanges)

(From Devinsky O, Feldmann E: Anatomy. p. 1. In Examination of the Cranial and Peripheral Nerves. Churchill Livingstone, New York, 1988, with permission.)

RATING SCALE FOR MOTOR STRENGTH*

Score	Examination
0	No muscular contraction
1	Flicker or trace of contraction
2	Movement with elimination of gravity
3	Movement against gravity
4	Movement against gravity with variable resistance
5	Movement with firm and maximal resistance several times

* The motor examination should also include bulk, abnormal movements, and tone in addition to strength.

DERMATOMES

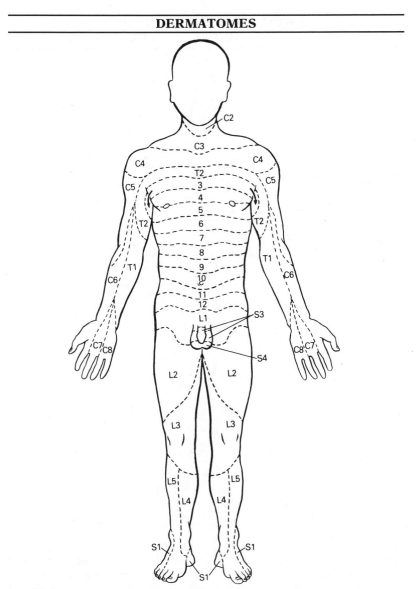

(Modified from Haymaker W, Woodhall B: Peripheral Nerve Injuries. WB Saunders, Philadelphia, 1953, p. 28, as in Devinsky O, Feldmann E: Anatomy. p. 1. In Examination of the Cranial and Peripheral Nerves, Churchill Livingstone, New York, 1988, with permission.)

CUTANEOUS FIELDS OF THE PERIPHERAL NERVES

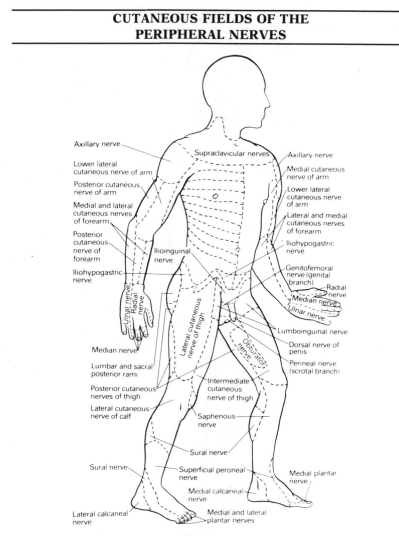

(Modified from Haymaker W, Woodhull B: Peripheral Nerve Injuries. WB Saunders, Philadelphia, 1953, p. 42, as in Devinsky O, Feldmann E: Anatomy. p. 1. In Examination of the Cranial and Peripheral Nerves. Churchill Livingstone, New York, 1988, with permission.)

CUTANEOUS FIELDS OF THE
PERIPHERAL NERVES (*Continued*)

I. Sensory modalities
   A. Primary
      1. Pain, temperture, light touch, vibration, position
   B. Cortical sensation
      1. Extinction, graphesthesia, stereognosis, two-point discrimination

COORDINATION/GAIT/STATION

I. Cerebellar testing
   A. Finger-nose test
   B. Rapid alternating movements for dysdiadochokinesia
   C. Rhythmic tapping with hand and/or foot
   D. Rebound test (impaired check)
   E. Heel-shin test
   F. Romberg's test
   G. Hypotonia
II. Gait: Testing of the gait should include observation of stability, foot placement (heel strike first contact with ground), width of stance, pelvic stability, axial posture, arm swing, and associated involuntary movements (e.g., dystonic postures)
   A. Normal gait
   B. Tandem gait

DEEP TENDON REFLEXES

Reflex	Roots*	Nerve
Jaw jerk	CN V	Mandibular division
Deltoid	**C5,** C6	Axillary
Pectoralis	C5–C8	Lateral and medial pectoral
Biceps	C5, C6	Musculocutaneous
Brachioradialis	C5, **C6**	Radial
Triceps	**C7,** C8	Radial
Hoffmann's reflex	C7, C8, T1	Median/ulnar
Knee	L2, **L3, L4**	Femoral
Hamstring	L5, **S1,** S2	Sciatic
Ankle	**S1,** S2	Tibial

* Boldface type signifies the major root contribution.

RELIABILITY OF SYMPTOMS, SIGNS, AND LABORATORY TESTS IN NEUROLOGY

Symptoms	Kappa*
TIA	0.65
Localization of TIA	0.36
Previous TIA	0.19
Previous stroke	0.40
Severe headache at onset of stroke	0.52
Signs	
Extensor plantar response	0.24
Asymmetric tendon reflexes	0.49
Inequality of pupils	0.61
Pupillary light response	0.64
Spontaneous eye movements	0.46
Oculocephalic responses	0.49
Motor response on Glasgow coma scale	0.66
Straight-leg raising	0.56
Hunt and Hess scale for subarachnoid hemorrhage	0.43
Neck stiffness	0.51
Sensory deficits	0.35
Visual fields	0.40
Ataxia	0.45
Neck bruit	0.67
Laboratory tests	
Abnormality on electroencephalogram	0.86
≥50% Stenosis on carotid angiogram	0.86
≥50% Stenosis on duplex scan of carotid	0.92
Normal CT scan in stroke patients	0.68
Small deep infarct on CT scan	0.76
Intracerebral hemorrhage on CT scan	1.0

* Kappa is a statistical measurement of reproducibility. In this case, a high kappa score means that two people examining the same patient are likely to agree. For example, two people reading a CT scan are very likely to agree about the presence of an intracerebral hemorrhage; the chances for agreement are much lower for the presence of an extensor plantar response.
(From Shinar D, Gross CR, Mohr JP, et al.: Interobserver variability in the assessment of neurologic history and examination in the Stroke Data Bank. Arch Neruol 42(6):557–565, 1985, with permission.)

4

DIFFERENTIAL DIAGNOSIS

Cranial Nerves

CN I—ANOSMIA

I. Age-related
II. Trauma (e.g., head injury, cranial surgery)
III. Heavy smoking
IV. Chronic rhinitis and sinusitis
V. Mucosal swelling (from hormonal and metabolic disorders)
VI. Overstimulation (temporary loss)
VII. Hysterical/malingering
VIII. Toxins (e.g., cocaine, amphetamine, lead, calcium)
IX. Frontal lobe masses (e.g., tumor, abscess)
X. Subarachnoid hemorrhage
XI. Infarct in anterior cerebral artery distribution
XII. Atrophic rhinitis (leprosy)
XIII. Local radiation therapy
XIV. Meningitis
XV. Infections (e.g., viral hepatitis, syphilis, influenza)
XVI. Osteomyelitis of frontal or ethmoid sinuses
XVII. Kallmann syndrome (congenital anosmia and hypogonadotropic hypogonadism)
XVIII. Albinism
XIX. Hydrocephalus
XX. Possibly multiple sclerosis
XXI. Possibly parkinsonism
XXII. Tumors of olfactory epithelium

CN II—OPTIC NEUROPATHY: LOCATIONS AND COMMON LESIONS

I. Ocular lesions
  A. Congenital (e.g., Coats disease)
  B. Trauma (hematoma, detached lens/retina)
  C. Inflammation
  D. Tumor (benign or malignant, primary or metastatic)
II. Optic nerve/sheath lesions
  A. Infection (e.g., tuberculosis)
  B. Inflammation (e.g., sarcoid)
  C. Demyelinating disease
  D. Vascular defect (e.g., ischemic optic neuropathy)
  E. Trauma
  F. Metabolic (e.g., Graves' disease)
  G. Drusen
  H. Tumor (e.g., glioma, meningioma)
  I. Miscellaneous (e.g., patulous CSF spaces)
III. Retrobulbar masses
  A. Bony orbit (e.g., fibrous dysplasia, metastases)
  B. Sinus, lacrimal gland lesions
  C. Tumors, tumor-like conditions (e.g., hemangioma/lymphangioma, dermoid, pseudotumor)
IV. Chiasmal lesions
  A. Vascular defect (aneurysm)
  B. Infection/inflammation (e.g., tuberculosis, sarcoid, exudative bacterial meningitis)
  C. Tumor (e.g., adenoma, glioma, meningioma, craniopharyngioma)
V. Retrochiasmal (brain parenchyma) lesions
  A. Vascular defect (e.g., infarct, vascular malformation)
  B. Infection/inflammation (e.g., multiple sclerosis, abscess)
  C. Hemorrhage
  D. Neoplasm (primary or metastatic)

(From Osborn AG, Harnsberger HR: MRI of cranial nerves. MRI Decisions 4:3–11, 1990, with permission.)

TRANSIENT MONOCULAR BLINDNESS

   I. Embolic
      A. Carotid bifurcation thromboembolism
      B. Great vessel or distal internal carotid atheroembolism
      C. Cardiogenic emboli (valve, mural thrombus, intracardiac tumor)
      D. Drug abuse-related intravascular emboli
  II. Hemodynamic
      A. Extensive atheromatous occlusive disease
      B. Inflammatory arteritis (Takayasu's disease)
      C. Hypoperfusion (e.g., cardiac failure, acute hypovolemia, coagulopathy, blood viscosity)
 III. Ocular
      A. Anterior ischemic optic neuropathy
      B. Central or branch retinal artery occlusion (often embolic)
      C. Central retinal vein occlusion
      D. Nonvascular causes (e.g., hemorrhage, pressure, tumor, congenital)
  IV. Neurologic
      A. Brainstem, vestibular, or oculomotor
      B. Optic neuritis, compression of optic nerve or chiasm
      C. Papilledema
      D. Multiple sclerosis
      E. Migraine
      F. Psychogenic
   V. Idiopathic

(From The Amaurosis Fugax Study Group: Current management of amaurosis fugax. Stroke 21:201–208, 1990, with permission.)

CN III—OCULOMOTOR PALSY

I. Intra-axial (midbrain)
   A. Ischemia
   B. Tumor
   C. Inflammation/demyelination
   D. Aneurysm
   E. Hemorrhage
   F. Tuberculoma
II. Subarachnoid space
   A. Aneurysm (usually posterior communicating; less commonly, posterior cerebral or superior cerebellar)
   B. Meningitis
   C. Uncal herniation
III. Cavernous sinus/superior orbital fissure
   A. Aneurysm (internal carotid)
   B. Tumor (meningioma, pituitary adenoma, metastatic)
   C. Tolosa-Hunt syndrome
   D. Cavernous sinus thrombosis
   E. Pituitary apoplexy
   F. Carotid-cavernous fistula
   G. Dural AVM
   H. Diabetic infarction of CN III (pupil spared in 80% of cases)
   I. Fungal infection
   J. Herpes zoster
IV. Orbit
   A. Orbital pseudotumor
   B. Orbital blowout fracture
V. Miscellaneous
   A. Guillain-Barré syndrome (Miller-Fisher variant)
   B. Migraine
   C. Arteritis
May be mimicked by:
   A. Internuclear ophthalmoplegia
   B. Myasthenia gravis
   C. Thyroid ophthalmopathy
   D. Skew deviation
   E. Brown superior oblique tendon sheath syndrome
   F. Strabismus

CN III—OCULOMOTOR PALSY (*Continued*)

Management of isolated third nerve palsies—an isolated third cranial nerve palsy is an important neurological sign. Although associated with cerebral aneurysms, angiography is not always indicated. The following guidelines should help the clinician to make the correct decision:

A. All patients under age 40–50 years should undergo CT or MRI, CSF examination, and angiography, regardless of the state of the pupil.

B. Patients over the age of 40–50 years with *pupillary-sparing* third nerve palsies need not undergo immediate angiography, but must be observed closely.

C. All patients over age 40–50 years presenting with isolated third nerve palsy *with* pupillary involvement should have CT or MRI, CSF examination, and angiography.

D. Ten to 20% of patients with ischemic third nerve palsies will have pupillary involvement, and thus result in negative angiograms in spite of the above guidelines. The dividing age (40–50 years old) varies with other risk factors that may predispose to neural ischemia, such as diabetes.

(From Burde RM, Savino PJ, Trobe JD: Diplopia. pp. 184–185. In Clinical Decisions in Neuro-ophthalmology. CV Mosby, St. Louis, 1985, with permission.)

CN IV—TROCHLEAR PALSY

I. Intra-axial
   A. Infarction
II. Subarachnoid space
   A. Trauma
   B. Meningitis
   C. Tumor (e.g., pinealoma, tentorial meningioma)
III. Cavernous sinus/superior orbital fissure
   A. Diabetic infarction
   B. Aneurysm
   C. Tumor (e.g., meningioma, pituitary adenoma, metastases)
   D. Tolosa-Hunt syndrome
   E. Cavernous sinus thrombosis
   F. Carotid-cavernous fistula
   G. Herpes zoster
IV. Mimics
   A. Myasthenia gravis
   B. Thyroid ophthalmopathy
   C. Skew deviation
   D. Strabismus

CN V—TRIGEMINAL NEUROPATHY

  I. Intra-axial (pons)
   A. Vascular
   B. Neoplastic
   C. Demyelination
   D. Syringobulbia
 II. Cerebellopontine angle
   A. Acoustic neuroma
   B. Trigeminal neuroma
   C. Subacute/chronic meningitis (see CP angle lesion list for additional causes)
III. Petrous apex
   A. Gradenigo petrositis
IV. Skull base/orbital fissure/cavernous sinus
   A. Nasopharyngeal tumors
   B. Metastatic carcinoma
   C. Trauma
 V. Miscellaneous
   A. Diabetes
   B. Systemic lupus erythematosus
   C. Scleroderma
   D. Systemic sclerosis
   E. Sjögren syndrome
   F. Trigeminal neuralgia
   G. Herpes (zoster and simplex)
   H. Trichloroethylene

CN VI—ABDUCENS PALSY

I. Intra-axial
   A. Infarction
   B. Möbius syndrome
   C. Duane retraction syndrome
   D. Wernicke-Korsakoff syndrome
II. Subarachnoid space
   A. Trauma
   B. Increased intracranial pressure
   C. Subarachnoid hemorrhage
   D. Basal meningitis
   E. Clivus tumor
   F. Large cerebellopontine angle masses (see separate list)
   G. Gradenigo syndrome (ipsilateral V and VI), petrositis
   H. Sarcoid
   I. Infiltration (e.g., lymphoma, leukemia, carcinoma)
III. Cavernous sinus/superior orbital fissure
   A. Aneurysm
   B. Tumor (e.g., meningioma, pituitary adenoma, nasopharyngeal carcinoma)
   C. Tolosa-Hunt syndrome
   D. Thrombosis
   E. Carotid-cavernous fistula
   F. Dural AVM
   G. Herpes zoster
IV. Miscellaneous
   A. Diabetic infarction
   B. Vasculopathic
   C. Following LP
   D. Parainfectious
May be mimicked by:
   A. Myasthenia gravis
   B. Thyroid ophthalmopathy
   C. Convergence spasm
   D. Congenital esotropia

CHRONIC PROGRESSIVE EXTERNAL OPHTHALMOPLEGIA (CPEO)*

    I. Myasthenia gravis
   II. Graves' ophthalmopathy
  III. Brainstem disease (Möbius syndrome, progressive supranuclear palsy)
  IV. Orbital pseudotumor
   V. Oculopharyngeal dystrophy
  VI. Kearns-Sayre syndrome
 VII. Myotubular myopathy
VIII. Stephens syndrome (CPEO, ataxia, peripheral neuropathy)
  IX. Myotonic dystrophy
   X. Abetalipoproteinemia (Bassen-Kornzweig syndrome)
  XI. Refsum's disease
 XII. Congenital extraocular fibrosis/adherence

* Paresis of extraocular movements, with sparing of pupillary function and accommodation.

CN VII—FACIAL PALSY

  I. Supranuclear
     A. Cerebral lesions (infarct, structural lesions)
     B. Progressive supranuclear palsy
 II. Nuclear/pontine
     A. Vascular
     B. Neoplasm
     C. Polioencephalitis
     D. Multiple sclerosis
     E. Syringobulbia
III. Cerebellopontine angle (see CP angle syndrome list)
IV. Facial canal
     A. Bell's palsy
     B. Skull fracture
     C. Mumps
     D. Scarlet fever
     E. Malaria
     F. Vascular insufficiency
     G. Otitis media
     H. Cholesteatoma
     I. Dermoid
     J. Lyme disease
 V. Geniculate ganglion
     A. Herpes zoster
VI. Extracranial
     A. Trauma
        1. Facial trauma
        2. Parotid surgery
        3. Mastoidopathy
        4. Leprosy

FACIAL DIPLEGIA

   I. Brainstem lesion
     A. Contusion
     B. Pontine infarction
     C. Tumor (glioma)
   II. Sarcoidosis (uveoparotid fever)
  III. Basilar meningitis
  IV. Lymphoma
   V. Polymyositis
  VI. Myasthenia gravis
 VII. Lyme disease
VIII. Guillain-Barré syndrome (Miller-Fisher variant)
  IX. Bilateral acoustic neuroma
   X. Bilateral Bell's palsy (rare)
  XI. Acute idiopathic polyneuritis
 XII. Melkersson-Rosenthal syndrome
XIII. Möbius syndrome
XIV. Myotonic dystrophy
 XV. Facioscapulohumeral dystrophy
XVI. Congenital myotonic dystrophy

DYSGEUSIA

    I. Heavy smoking (especially cigar smoking)
   II. Dryness of the mouth (xerostomia)
  III. Cranial irradiation
  IV. Pandysautonomia
   V. Influenza
  VI. Scleroderma
 VII. Acute hepatitis
VIII. Viral encephalitis
  IX. Myxedema
   X. Systemic malignancy
  XI. Deficiency of vitamins B_{12} and A
 XII. Zinc deficiency
XIII. Drugs
     A. Griseofulvin
     V. Amitriptyline
     C. Thyroid medications
     D. Chlorambucil
     E. Cholestyramine
     F. Penicillamine
     G. Procarbazine
     H. Vincristine
     I. Vinblastine
XIV. Unilateral loss
     A. Bell's palsy
     B. Unilateral lesions of the medulla
     C. Unilateral lesions of the thalamus and parietal cortex

TINNITUS

I. Subjective (heard only by patient)
   A. Physiological tinnitus (present in 80–90% of normal individuals, in soundproof rooms)
   B. Disorders of external ear or jaw
      1. Cerumen
      2. TMJ disease
   C. Disorders of middle ear
      1. Otosclerosis
      2. Otitis media
   D. Disorders of inner ear/eighth nerve
      1. Presbycusis
      2. Following high-intensity sound
      3. Head trauma
      4. Menière's disease
      5. CP angle tumors
      6. Glomus tumors
      7. Syphilis
   E. Pontine lesions (complex auditory illusions)
   F. Ototoxic drugs (see Vertigo)
   G. Systemic disorders
      1. Fever
      2. Hypertension
      3. Anemia
      4. Tobacco
      5. Ethanol
   H. Miscellaneous
      1. Elevated intracranial pressure*
      2. Intracranial neoplasms*
      3. Venous sinus thrombosis*
      4. Intracranial aneurysms*
      5. Meningioma of the middle ear*
II. Objective (may be heard by examiner)
   A. Abnormally patent eustachian tube—blowing
   B. Palatal myoclonus
   C. AVM (most commonly dural)*
   D. Carotid stenosis or occlusion* (atherosclerotic, dissection, or fibro-muscular dyplasia)
   E. Glomus tympanicum tumor*
   F. Venous hum
   G. Arteriovenous shunts*

List Continues

TINNITUS (*Continued*)

H. Aortic valvular disease*
I. Increased cardiac output*
J. Vascular neoplasms of the middle ear*
K. Possibly asymmetry of the jugular bulbs*

* May be associated with pulsatile tinnitus.

(Modified from Ruff RC: Auditory and vestibular disturbances. pp. 119–120. In Swanson PD: Signs & Symptoms in Neurology. JB Lippincott, Philadelphia, 1984, with permission.)

VERTIGO

I. Central
  A. Brainstem TIA/infarct (e.g., Wallenberg syndrome)
  B. Posterior fossa tumors/masses
  C. Multiple sclerosis
  D. Cerebellar hemorrhage
  E. Temporal lobe epilepsy
  F. Syringobulbia
  G. Arnold-Chiari deformity
  H. Basilar migraine
II. Peripheral
  A. Physiological (e.g., motion sickness)
  B. Benign positional vertigo
  C. Menière's disease
  D. Labyrinthitis
  E. Vestibular neuronitis
  F. Perilymph fistula
  G. Drugs/toxins
    1. Alcohol
    2. Phenytoin
    3. Phenobarbital
    4. Carbamazepine
    5. Primidone
    6. Furosemide
    7. Ethacrynic acid
    8. Aminoglycosides
    9. Salicylates
    10. Quinine
    11. Quinidine
    12. Antineoplastics (e.g., cisplatin, nitrogen mustard)
    13. Heavy metals (e.g., mercury, gold, lead, arsenic)
  H. Posttraumatic

FEATURES OF PERIPHERAL AND CENTRAL VERTIGO

	Peripheral	Central
Nystagmus	Unidirectional, associated with nystagmus	Vertical nystagmus usually implies a central lesion; with horizontal gaze, often changes with direction of gaze
Nystagmus latency	Latency before onset; transient (<1 min)	No latency; persistent (>1 min)
Caloric response	Decreased on the side of the lesion	Normal
Description of vertigo	Severe, often rotational	Mild
Nausea and vomiting	Usually present	Usually absent
Hearing loss, tinnitus	Frequently present	Absent
Cranial nerve or brainstem signs	Absent	Often present
Tendency to fall	Often falls to the side opposite the nystagmus (direction of fast component)	Often falls to the side of the lesion
Visual fixation	Inhibits nystagmus and vertigo	No change

HEARING LOSS

I. Infarction of internal auditory artery
II. Hereditary
III. Viral infections
  A. Mumps
  B. Measles
  C. Mononucleosis
IV. Meningitis
V. Drugs
  A. Aminoglycosides
  B. Chloramphenicol
  C. Chloroquine
  D. Furosemide
  E. Ethacrynic acid
  F. Acetylsalicylic acid
  G. Quinine
  H. Quinidine
  I. Cisplatin
  J. Nitrogen mustard
  K. Mercury
  L. Gold
  M. Lead
  N. Arsenic
VI. Otosclerosis (usually autosomal dominant)
VII. Acoustic trauma (sustained loud noises)
VIII. Fractures of the temporal bone
IX. Hypothyroidism
X. Chronic otitis
XI. Neoplastic disorders
XII. Menière's disease
XIII. Multiple sclerosis (involving cochlear nerve fibers)
XIV. Cerebellopontine angle tumors (see separate list)
  A. Schwannoma
  B. Meningioma
  C. Cholesteatoma
  D. Lymphoma
XV. Congenital (rubella during pregnancy)
XVI. External canal occlusion (e.g., cerumen)

CN IX, X, and XI—NEUROPATHY

I. Brainstem
   A. Stroke (Wallenberg lateral medullary syndrome)
   B. Hemorrhage (hypertensive, AVM)
   C. Multiple sclerosis
   D. Tumor (glioma, metastases)
II. Cistern/jugular foramen
   A. Infection
      1. Meningitis
      2. Malignant external otitis
   B. Vascular malformation
      1. Vertebrobasilar dolichoectasia
      2. Aneurysm (vertebral artery)
      3. Jugular vein thrombosis
   C. Tumor
      1. Paraganglioma
      2. Neural (e.g., schwannoma, neurofibroma)
      3. Squamous cell carcinoma (nasopharynx, oropharynx), direct extension
      4. Non-Hodgkin's lymphoma
      5. Minor salivary gland
      6. Metastases to skull base
      7. Rhabdomyosarcoma (children)
   D. Trauma
      1. Penetrating wounds
      2. Surgical wounds (e.g., radical neck dissection)

CN IX, X, and XI—NEUROPATHY (*Continued*)

III. Distal (vagal neuropathy only)
- A. Vascular
  1. Arch aneurysm on left
  2. Jugular vein thrombosis
- B. Infection
  1. Carotid space
  2. Mediastinum
- C. Surgical trauma
  1. Thyroidectomy
- D. Tumor
  1. Paraganglioma, neuroma
  2. Primary or nodular squamous cell carcinoma, other metastases
  3. Thyroid malignancies
  4. Lymphoma
  5. Lung carcinoma, other mediastinal masses (on left)

(From Osborn AG, Harnsberger HR: MRI of cranial nerves. MRI Decisions 5:2–15, 1990, with permission.)

CN XII—HYPOGLOSSAL NEUROPATHY

I. Brainstem
  A. Stroke
  B. Hemorrhage
  C. Multiple sclerosis
  D. Bulbar-type polio
  E. Tumor (glioma)
  F. Syringobulbia
  G. Botulism
II. Subanachnoid/cisternal
  A. Vertebrobasilar dolichoectasia
  B. Aneurysm, subarachnoid hemorrhage
  C. Skull base tumors (e.g., chordoma, meningioma)
  D. Basilar invagination
  E. Basilar meningitis
  F. Arnold-Chiari malformation
III. Base of skull
  A. Trauma
  B. Neoplasm (metastases, primary bone tumor, squamous cell carcinoma, schwannoma/neuroma, glomus, meningioma)
  C. Infection (mucormycosis, Pseudomonas sp; malignant external otitis)
IV. Nasopharynx, carotid space
  A. Squamous cell carcinoma, non-Hodgkin's lymphoma, metastases, glomus tumors
  B. Infection
  C. Trauma
  D. Vascular thrombosis
  E. Ectasia
V. Sublingual
  A. Squamous cell carcinoma
  B. Abscess

(From Osborn AG, Harnsberger HR: MRI of cranial nerves. MRI Decisions 5:2–15, 1990, with permission.)

BRAINSTEM AND CRANIAL NERVE SYNDROMES

Syndrome	Location	Cranial Nerves Involved	Tracts and Nuclei Involved	Signs
Weber	Base of midbrain	III	Corticospinal tract.	Oculomotor palsy with contralateral hemiparesis.
Claude	Tegmentum of midbrain	III	Red nucleus and brachium conjunctivum.	Oculomotor palsy, contralateral ataxia and tremor.
Benedikt	Tegmentum of midbrain	III	Red nucleus, corticospinal tract, and brachium conjunctivum.	Oculomotor palsy with contralateral hemiparesis, ataxia, and tremor.
Nothnagel	Tectum of midbrain	Unilateral or bilateral III	Superior cerebellar peduncles.	Ocular palsies and cerebellar ataxia.
Parinaud	Dorsal midbrain		Supranuclear mechanism of upward gaze, posterior commissure, periaqueductal gray.	Paralysis of upward, occasionally downward gaze, paralysis of accommodation, unreactive pupils, ocular divergence.
Internuclear ophthalmoplegia (INO)	Pontine or midbrain tegmentum		Medial longitudinal fasciculus.	Ipsilateral adduction palsy or slowed adduction saccade, preseved convergence, contralateral monocular nystagmus.
One-and-a-half	Pontine tegmentum		Medial longitudinal fasciculus, pontine gaze center.	INO with contralateral gaze palsy.
Millard-Gubler	Basis pontis	VII, often VI	Corticospinal tract.	Lower motor neuron facial weakness, contralateral hemiparesis, abducens or gaze palsy to side of lesion.
Wallenberg (lateral medullary)	Lateral tegmentum of medulla	Spinal V, IX, X, XI	Lateral spinothalamic tract, descending pupillodilator fibers,	Ipsilateral: V, IX, X, XI palsy, central Horner syndrome, cerebellar

List Continues

BRAINSTEM AND CRANIAL NERVE SYNDROMES (*Continued*)

Syndrome	Location	Cranial Nerves Involved	Tracts and Nuclei Involved	Signs
			spinocerebellar and olivocerebellar tracts.	ataxia; contralateral loss of pain and temperature sense (see separate list).
Lateral pontomedullary syndrome	Lateral tegmentum of medulla and pons	Spinal V, VII, VII, IX, X, XI	As with lateral medullary syndrome.	Findings of lateral medullary syndrome plus ipsilateral facial weakness and hearing disturbance.
Dejerine's anterior bulbar syndrome	Medial medulla	XII	Ipsilateral pyramid and medial lemniscus.	Contralateral hemiplegia and loss of position and vibration sense.
Foix	Sphenoidal fissure	III, IV, V_1, VI		
Tolosa-Hunt	Lateral wall of cavernous sinus	III, IV, V_1, V_2, VI		
Jacod	Retrosphenoidal space	II, III, IV, V, VI		
Gradenigo	Petrous apex	V, VI		
Vernet	Cerebellopontine angle	V, VII, VIII, occasionally IX		
Collet-Sicard	Jugular foramen	IX, X, XI		
	Posterior laterocondylar space	IX, X, XI, XIII		
Villaret, Mackenzie	Posterior retroparotid space	IX, X, XI, XII and Horner syndrome		
Tapia	Posterior retroparotid space	IX, XII ± XI		

Neurological Symptoms and Syndromes

TRANSIENT NEUROLOGICAL SYNDROMES AND THEIR COMMON CAUSES

Transient Neurological Symptom	Common Causes
Loss of consciousness	Seizure disorder
	Vertebrobasilar ischemia
	Metabolic encephalopathy
	Cardiac abnormality
	Autonomic dysfunction
Alteration of sensorium or confusion	Vertebrobasilar ischemia
	Seizure disorder
	Dominant hemispheric lesion
	Multiple sclerosis
	Cardiovascular disturbance
	Metabolic encephalopathy
	Endocrine dysfunction
Limb weakness	Cerebral hemispheric dysfunction
	Internal carotid artery lesion
	Posterior cerebral artery lesion
	Multiple sclerosis
	Spinal cord dysfunction
	Muscle weakness disorders
Amnesia	Seizure disorder
	Transient global amnesia
	Posterior cerebral artery disease
Tonic-clonic jerks	Seizure disorder
	Hysteria
Drop attacks	Cerebral ischemia
	Cardiac abnormality
	Cataplexy
Diplopia and/or intense headaches	Intracranial aneurysm
	Arteriovenous malformation
	Space-occupying lesion
Vertigo	Labyrinthine disease
	Vertebrobasilar disease
	Seizure disorder
Behavioral abnormalities	Seizure disorder
	Alcohol abuse
	Transient global amnesia
	Hypothalamic disease

(From Gnanamuthu C: Transient neurological symptoms. Postgrad Med 87:99–119, 1990, with permission.)

APHASIAS

Syndrome	Fluency	Repetition	Comprehension	Classical Localization
Broca's aphasia	Poor	Impaired	Good	Dominant premotor cortex (Brodman's area 44)
Wernicke's aphasia	Good	Impaired	Very poor	Posterior portion of superior dominant temporal gyrus
Conduction aphasia	Good	Poor	Good	Supramarginal gyrus and arcuate fasciculus; or insula, auditory cortex, and underlying white matter
Global aphasia	Poor	Poor	Poor	Extensive damage to language areas in dominant cortex
Transcortical motor aphasia	Poor	Good	Good	Border zone between major arteries (anterior)
Transcortical sensory aphasia	Good	Good	Poor	Border zone between major arteries (posterior)
Isolation of speech area	Poor	Good	Poor	Border zone between major arteries (extensive)
Anomic aphasia	Good but with word-finding pauses	Good	Good	Second and third temporal gyrus; many other areas, nonspecific sign
Alexia without agraphia	Good	Good	Good	Posterior corpus callosum and left occipital lobe
Alexia with agraphia	Good	Good	Good	Left inferior parietal (angular gyrus)
Pure word deafness	Good	Poor	Absent	Bilateral deep temporal lesions

AMNESTIC SYNDROMES

Syndrome	Characteristics	Common Causes	Prognosis
Acute confusional state	Retrograde and anterograde amnesia, disordered attention and thought, abnormal EEG	Drugs, toxins, infections, metabolic, trauma	Usually reversible
Transient global amnesia	Retrograde amnesia for finite period, rapid onset and recovery, EEG usually normal	Etiology unknown, ?vascular, ?epileptic	Reversible
Temporal lobe seizures	Retrograde amnesia for finite period, rapid onset, EEG shows discharge focus	Epileptic	Reversible
Wernicke-Korsakoff	Confusion, anterograde amnesia, unaware of deficits, confabulation	Alcoholism, thiamine deficiency	Some recovery, often residual deficits
Hippocampal amnesia	Failure to form new memories, relatively intact cognition otherwise	Bilateral mesial temporal lesions, herpes simplex encephalitis, trauma	Some recovery, often residual deficits
Benign senescent forgetfulness	Forget trivial facts	Aging	Slowly progressive
Dementia	Global retrograde and anterograde amnesia, initial impairment of memory and learning	See separate classification	Progressive

DEMENTIA

I. Vascular
   A. Multi-infarct
   B. Binswanger's disease
II. Structural
   A. Hydrocephalus (increased pressure)
   B. Normal pressure hydrocephalus
   C. Intracranial tumors
   D. Chronic subdural
III. Myelin
   A. Multiple sclerosis
   B. Leukodystrophies (also under inherited disorders)
   C. Marchiafava-Bignami syndrome
IV. Metabolic
   A. Hypothyroidism
   B. Wernicke-Korsakoff syndrome
   C. Hepatic encephalopathy
   D. Uremia
   E. Vitamin B_{12} deficiency
   F. Nicotinic acid deficiency (pellagra)
   G. Electrolytes (e.g., hypercalcemia)
   H. Drugs
   I. Toxins
      1. Alcohol
      2. Lead
      3. Carbon monoxide

DEMENTIA (*Continued*)

V. Infectious
  A. Creutzfeldt-Jakob disease
  B. Progressive multifocal leukoencephalopathy
  C. Syphilis
  D. Chronic meningitis (fungal, tuberculous)
  E. Subacute sclerosing panencephalitis
  F. HIV
  G. Whipple's disease
VI. Neurodegenerative
  A. Alzheimer's disease
  B. Pick's disease
  C. Huntington's disease
  D. Parkinson's disease/Shy-Drager syndrome
  E. Progressive supranuclear palsy
  F. Olivopontocerebellar atrophy
  G. Familial dementia with spastic paraparesis
  H. Parkinson-ALS-dementia complex of Guam
VII. Neoplastic
  A. Meningeal carcinomatosis
  B. Limbic encephalitis
VIII. Inherited neurometabolic disorder
  A. Wilson's disease
  B. Krabbe's globoid body leukodystrophy
  C. Metachromatic leukodystrophy
  D. Adult neuronal ceroid-lipofuscinosis (Kufs disease)
IX. Seizure
  A. Epilepsy
X. Trauma
  A. Posttraumatic
  B. ?Radiation
XI. Psychogenic/psychiatric
  A. Depression, pseudodementia

ORGANIC CAUSES OF DELIRIUM

I. Intoxication
   A. Alcohol: ethyl and methyl
   B. Drugs: anticholinergic agents, sedative hypnotics, digitalis derivatives, opiates, corticosteroids, salicylates, antibiotics, anticonvulsants, antiarrhythmic and antihypertensive drugs, antineoplastic agents, cimetidine, lithium, antiparkinson agents, disulfiram, indomethacin
   C. Inhalants: gasoline, glue, ether, nitrous oxide, nitrates
   D. Toxins
      1. Industrial: carbon disulfide, organic solvents, methylchloride and bromide, heavy metals, organophosphorus insecticides, carbon monoxide
      2. Plants and mushrooms
      3. Venoms (e.g., snakebite)
II. Withdrawal syndromes
   A. Alcohol (delirium tremens)
   B. Sedative/hypnotics: barbiturates, chloral hydrate, chlordiazepoxide, diazepam, ethchlorvynol, glutethimide, meprobamate, methyprylon, paraldehyde
   C. Amphetamines
III. Metabolic disorders
   A. Hypoxia
   B. Hypoglycemia
   C. Hepatic, renal, pancreatic, pulmonary insufficiency (encephalopathy)
   D. Errors of metabolism: porphyria, carcinoid syndrome, hepatolenticular degeneration (Wilson's disease)

ORGANIC CAUSES OF DELIRIUM (*Continued*)

IV. Nutritional disorders
  A. Avitaminosis: nicotinic acid, thiamine, cyanocobalamin (vitamin B_{12}), folate, pyridoxine
  B. Hypervitaminosis: intoxication by vitamins A and D
  C. Disorders of fluid and electrolyte metabolism: dehydration, water intoxication, alkalosis, acidosis, hypernatremia, hyponatremia, hypercalcemia, hypocalcemia, hypermagnesemia, hypomagnesemia
 V. Hormonal disorders
  A. Hyperinsulinism, hyperthyroidism, hypothyroidism, hypopituitarism, Addison's disease, Cushing syndrome, hypoparathyroidism, hyperparathyroidism
VI. Infections
  A. Systemic: pneumonia, typhoid, typhus, acute rheumatic fever, malaria, influenza, mumps, diphtheria, brucellosis, infectious mononucleosis, infectious hepatitis, malaria, subacute bacterial endocarditis, bacteremia, septicemia, Rocky Mountain spotted fever, legionnaire's disease
  B. Intracranial (acute, subacute, and chronic): viral encephalitis, aseptic meningitis, rabies, herpes; bacterial meningitis—meningococcal, pneumococcal, *Haemophilus influenzae*, etc.; granulomatous angiitis
VII. Neoplasms
  A. Metastasis
  B. Remote effects

(From Massey EW, Coffey CE: Delirium: diagnosis and treatment. South Med J 76:1147–1150, 1983, with permission.)

EPISODIC WEAKNESS

  - I. Multiple sclerosis
 - II. Cerebral ischemia
- III. Periodic paralysis
   - A. Familial/hypokalemic
   - B. Hyperthyroid and periodic paralysis
   - C. Hyperkalemic
   - D. Congential paramyotonia
 - IV. Alcoholic myopathies
  - V. Myasthenia gravis
 - VI. Eaton-Lambert syndrome
- VII. Chronic relapsing polyneuropathy
- VIII. Atonic seizures
 - IX. Cataplexy
  - X. Other derangements of potassium homeostasis

INVOLUNTARY MOVEMENTS OF MUSCLE

Movement	Description
Fasciculation	Random contractions of groups of muscle fibers (visible as small twitches beneath the skin)
Myokymia	Rhythmic, undulating contractions of groups of muscle fibers
Cramp	Hard, painful contraction of one muscle
Myoclonus	Random, single, shock-like contractions of muscles
Ballism	Wild, forceful flinging of a limb (usually the arm)
Chorea	Random, brief, repetitive contractions of muscles
Athetosis	Contractions of muscles that cause writhing movements
Dystonia	Continuous contraction of opposing groups of muscles
Tremor	Rhythmic contractions of muscles
Partial motor seizure	Coarse, semirhythmic contractions of groups of muscles
Tics	Stereotyped, complex, repetitive movement

(Modified from Evans OB: Neurologic examination. p. 31. In Manual of Child Neurology. Churchill Livingstone, New York, 1987, with permission.)

MYOCLONUS

I. Physiologic
   A. Sleep jerks
   B. Anxiety
   C. Exercise
   D. Hiccup
   E. Benign infantile myoclonus with feeding
II. Essential (no known cause, no other neurological abnormality)
   A. Hereditary
   B. Benign, may be autosomal dominant
   C. Nocturnal myoclonus/periodic jerking during sleep
III. Vascular
   A. Post-stroke
IV. Structural
   A. Tumor
   B. Palatal myoclonus (lesions of Mollaret's triangle: inferior olive, dentate nucleus, red nucleus)
   C. Spinal cord lesions (segmental/spinal myoclonus)
V. Myelin
   A. Postinfectious
VI. Metabolic
   A. Postanoxia (Lance-Adams syndrome)
   B. Hepatic encephalopathy
   C. Uremia
   D. Dialysis syndrome
   E. Hyponatremia
   F. Hypoglycemia
   G. Hyperglycemia
   H. Drugs
      1. Tricyclic antidepressants
      2. Dopamine agonists
   I. Toxins
      1. Bismuth
      2. Heavy metals
      3. Methyl bromide
      4. DDT
VII. Infectious
   A. Creutzfeldt-Jakob disease
   B. Subacute sclerosing panencephalitis
   C. Encephalitis lethargica
   D. Arbovirus encephalitis
   E. Herpes simplex type I

List Continues

MYOCLONUS (*Continued*)

VIII. Neurodegenerative
    A. Parkinson's disease
    B. Alzheimer's disease
    C. Torsion dystonia
    D. Dentatorubral degeneration of Ramsay Hunt
    E. Friedreich's ataxia
    F. Ataxia-telangiectasia
    G. Progressive supranuclear palsy
    H. Huntington's disease
    I. Corticobasal ganglionic degeneration

IX. Paraneoplastic
    A. Opsoclonus-myoclonus

X. Inherited neurometabolic disorder
    A. Wilson's disease
    B. Hallervorden-Spatz disease
    C. Lafora body disease
    D. GM_2 gangliosidosis
    E. Gaucher's disease
    F. Krabbe's globoid body leukodystrophy
    G. Infantile neuronal ceroid-lipofuscinosis (Santavuori-Haltia disease)
    H. Juvenile neuronal ceroid-lipofuscinosis (Spielmeyer-Vogt or Batten's disease)
    I. Adult neuronal ceroid-lipofuscinosis (Kufs disease)
    J. Cherry-red spot myoclonus syndrome (type I)

XI. Epileptic myoclonus (seizures dominate, initially no encephalopathy)
    (EMG burst length: epileptic, 10–50 ms; nonepileptic, 50–300 ms)
    A. Fragments of epilepsy
    B. Childhood myoclonic epilepsies
    C. Benign familial myoclonic epilepsy
    D. Progressive myoclonus epilepsy (see separate classification)

XII. Trauma
    A. Posttraumatic
    B. Heat stroke
    C. Electric shock
    D. Decompression injury
    E. Postthalamotomy

XIII. Psychogenic

(Modified from Weiner WJ, Lang AE: Movement Disorders: A Comprehensive Survey. Futura Publishing, Mount Kisco, NY, 1989, with permission.)

HEMICHOREA/HEMIBALLISMUS

I. Vascular
- A. Infarction of caudate, striatum, lenticular, subthalamic nucleus
- B. TIA
- C. CNS lupus
- D. Subarachnoid hemorrhage

II. Structural
- A. Metastatic tumor
- B. AVM
- C. Venous angioma

III. Myelin
- A. Multiple sclerosis

IV. Metabolic
- A. Hyperglycemia
- B. Oral contraceptives
- C. Estrogens
- D. Phenytoin
- E. Neuroleptics
- F. L-dopa

V. Infectious
- A. AIDS
- B. Cerebral toxoplasmosis
- C. Tuberculous meningitis

VI. Trauma
- A. Thalamotomy
- B. Head trauma

(Modified from Dewey JRB, Jankovic J: Hemiballism-hemichorea. Arch Neurol 46:862–867, 1989, with permission.)

CHOREA

I. Vascular
   A. Infarct (hemichorea)
   B. Migraine
   C. Polycythemia
   D. Lupus
II. Structural
   A. Tumor, AVM (usually hemichorea)
III. Myelin
   A. Demyelination
   B. Pelizaeus-Merzbacher disease
IV. Metabolic
   A. Endocrine
      1. Hyperthyroidism
      2. Hypocalcemia
      3. Hypoparathyroidism with basal ganglia calcification
      4. Pregnancy
      5. Hyponatremia, hypernatremia
      6. Hypomagnesemia
      7. Hypoglycemia, hyperglycemia
   B. Drugs
      1. L-dopa and other dopamine agonists
      2. Neuroleptics
      3. Anticholinergics
      4. Tricyclic antidepressants
      5. Phenytoin, carbamazepine, phenobarbital, ethosuximide
      6. Pemoline
      7. Amphetamines
      8. Lithium
      9. Oral contraceptives
      10. Steroids
      11. Opiates
   C. Toxins
      1. Ethanol
      2. Kernicterus
      3. Mercury poisoning
      4. Manganese poisoning
      5. Thallium poisoning
      6. Carbon monoxide poisoning
      7. Toluene

CHOREA (*Continued*)

    D. Organ failure
       1. Anoxia
       2. Uremia
       3. Hepatic encephalopathy
       4. Hepatocerebral degeneration
    E. Nutritional
       1. Nicotinic acid deficiency (pellagra)
       2. Vitamin B_{12} (cobalamin) deficiency
       3. Vitamin B_1 (thiamin) deficiency
       4. Niacin deficiency
    F. Porphyria
    G. Mastocytosis
  V. Infectious
    A. Sydenham's chorea
    B. Lyme disease
    C. Encephalitis lethargica
    D. Creutzfeldt-Jakob disease
 VI. Neurodegenerative
    A. Huntington's disease
    B. Senile chorea
    C. Benign hereditary chorea
    D. Olivopontocerebellar atrophy
    E. Paroxysmal kinesogenic chorea/dystonia
    F. Ataxia-telangiectasia
    G. Azorean disease
    H. Neuroacanthocytosis
     I. Fahr's familial idiopathic basal ganglia calcification
    J. Dentato-rubro-pallido-luysian atrophy
    K. Juvenile neuroaxonal dystrophy
 VII. Inherited neurometabolic disorder
    A. Wilson's disease
    B. Hallervorden-Spatz disease
    C. Tuberous sclerosis
    D. Adult neuronal ceroid-lipofuscinosis (Kufs disease)
    E. Lesch-Nyhan syndrome
    F. Niemann-Pick disease
    G. Subacute necrotizing encephalomyelopathy (Leigh's disease)
VIII. Trauma
    A. Concussion
    B. Subdural hematoma
    C. Epidural hematoma

DYSTONIA

I. Primary
  A. Dystonia musculorum deformans/generalized dystonia
  B. Focal dystonias
    1. Cranial dystonias: Meigs syndrome, blepharospasm, oromandibular
    2. Spasmodic torticollis
    3. Writer's cramp and other occupational dystonias
    4. Spasmodic dystonia
    5. Others
  C. Idiopathic paroxysmal dystonias
    1. Paroxysmal kinesogenic chorea/dystonia
    2. Paroxysmal nonkinesogenic dystonia
II. Secondary
  A. Vascular
    1. Infarction
  B. Structural (usually causes hemidystonia)
    1. Tumor
    2. AVM
    3. Thalamotomy
    4. Brainstem lesion
  C. Myelin
    1. Multiple sclerosis
    2. Postinfectious demyelination
    3. Pelizaeus-Merzbacher disease
  D. Metabolic
    1. Anoxia
    2. Hypoparathyroidism with basal ganglia calcification
    3. Drugs
      a. Dopamine (D_2) antagonists
        (1) Acute dystonic reaction
        (2) Tardive dystonia
      b. L-dopa
      c. Ergot preparations
      d. Anticonvulsants (rarely)
      e. Neuroleptics
      f. Metoclopramide
    4. Toxins
      a. Reye syndrome
      b. Manganese poisoning
      c. Carbon monoxide poisoning

DYSTONIA (*Continued*)

      d. Carbon disulfide poisoning
      e. Methanol poisoning
      f. Kernicterus
E. Infectious
    1. Encephalitis lethargica
    2. Subacute sclerosing panencephalitis
    3. Wasp sting encephalopathy
F. Neurodegenerative
    1. Parkinson's disease (idiopathic)
    2. Progressive supranuclear palsy
    3. Olivopontocerebellar atrophy
    4. Huntington's disease
    5. Fahr's familial idiopathic basal ganglia calcification
    6. Dystonia-parkinsonism, L-dopa responsive
    7. Neuroacanthocytosis
    8. Pallidal degenerations
    9. Ataxia-telangiectasia
   10. Azorean disease
   11. Intraneuronal inclusion disease
   12. Rett syndrome
   13. Corticobasal ganglionic degeneration
   14. Dystonic amyotrophy
   15. Familial amyotrophic dystonic paraplegia
G. Inherited neurometabolic disorder
    1. Lysosomal storage
      a. Juvenile neuronal ceroid-lipofuscinosis (Spielmeyer-Vogt or Batten's disease)
      b. Adult neuronal ceroid-lipofuscinosis (Kufs disease)
      c. Metachromatic leukodystrophy
      d. GM_1 gangliosidosis
      e. GM_2 gangliosidosis
      f. Niemann-Pick disease
    2. Amino/organic acid
      a. Glutaric acidemia type I
      b. Hartnup's disease
      c. Homocystinuria
      d. Lesch-Nyhan syndrome
      e. Methylmalonic aciduria
    3. Mitochondrial encephalomyopathy
      a. Subacute necrotizing encephalomyelopathy (Leigh's disease)

List Continues

DYSTONIA (*Continued*)
---

    4. Metals
       a. Wilson's disease (copper)
       b. Hallervorden-Spatz disease (iron)
    5. Triose phosphate isomerase deficiency
  H. Trauma
    1. Head trauma
    2. Cervical cord injury
  I. Psychogenic dystonia

(Modified from Weiner WJ, Lang AE: Movement Disorders: A Comprehensive Survey. Futura Publishing, Mount Kisco, New York, 1989, with permission.)

TREMOR

I. Rest tremor
   A. Parkinson's disease
   B. Other parkinsonian syndromes (less commonly)
   C. Rubral tremor (rest < postural < intention)
   D. Wilson's disease
   E. Hepatocerebral degeneration
   F. Essential tremor (severe)
II. Postural and action ("terminal") tremor
   A. Physiological tremor
   B. Exaggerated physiological tremor
      1. Stress, fatigue, anxiety, emotion
      2. Endocrine
         a. Hypoglycemia
         b. Hyperthyroidism
         c. Pheochromocytoma
         d. Steroids (Cushing's syndrome, iatrogenic)
      3. Drugs
         a. Caffeine
         b. Beta agonists
         c. Theophylline
         d. Dopamine agonists
         e. Amphetamines
         f. Lithium
         g. Tricyclic antidepressants
         h. Neuroleptics
         i. Valproic acid
      4. Toxins
         a. Ethanol
         b. Mercury poisoning
         c. Lead poisoning
         d. Arsenic poisoning
   C. Essential tremor
   D. Primary writing tremor
   E. Associated with other CNS disorders
      1. Parkinson's disease
      2. Idiopathic/focal dystonias
      3. Other akinetic/rigid syndromes (see separate list)
   F. Associated with peripheral neuropathy
      1. Roussy-Lévy syndrome (Charcot-Marie-Tooth disease and tremor)
      2. Other neuropathies
   G. Cerebellar tremor

List Continues

TREMOR (*Continued*)

III. Intention tremor: disease of cerebellar outflow (dentate nucleus/superior cerebellar peduncle)
   A. Vascular
   B. Myelin
      1. Multiple sclerosis
   C. Metabolic
      1. Hepatocerebral degeneration
   D. Inherited neurometabolic disorder
      1. Wilson's disease
   E. Trauma
   F. Drugs/toxins
      1. Mercury poisoning
      2. Others
IV. Miscellaneous rhythmical movement disorders
   A. Psychogenic
   B. Rhythmic movements in dystonia (dystonic tremor, "myorhythmia")
   C. Rhythmical myoclonus
      1. Palatal myoclonus
      2. Branchial myoclonus
      3. Spinal myoclonus
   D. Asterixis
   E. Clonus
   F. Epilepsia partialis continua
   G. Hereditary chin quivering
   H. Spasmus nutans
   I. Head bobbing with third ventricular cysts
   J. Nystagmus

(From Weiner WJ, Lang AE: Movement Disorders: A Comprehensive Survey. Futura Publishing, New York, 1989, with permission.)

ATAXIA*

I. Vascular
   A. Stroke
   B. Migraine
II. Structural
   A. Tumor
   B. Cerebellar hemorrhage
   C. AVM
   D. Abscess
   E. Cyst (e.g., arachnoid, dermoid)
   F. Paget's disease
   G. Arnold-Chiari malformation
   H. Dandy-Walker cyst
   I. Basilar invagination/impression
   J. Posterior fossa subdural hematoma
III. Myelin
   A. Multiple sclerosis
   B. Pelizaeus-Merzbacher disease
   C. Other demyelination (e.g., postinfectious)
IV. Metabolic
   A. Toxins
      1. Ethanol
      2. Dilantin or other anticonvulsants
      3. Mercury poisoning
   B. Wernicke-Korsakoff syndrome
   C. Hypothyroidism
   D. Hepatic encephalopathy
   E. Vitamin E deficiency
V. Infectious
   A. Viral/postinfectious (commonly in children)
   B. Creutzfeldt-Jakob disease/kuru
   C. Gerstmann-Straussler syndrome
   D. Subacute sclerosing panencephalitis
VI. Neurodegenerative
   A. Olivopontocerebellar atrophy
   B. Friedreich's ataxia
   C. Dentatorubral degeneration of Ramsay Hunt (probably a variety of diseases, including mitochondrial, neurometabolic, and multisystem atrophies)
   D. Ataxia-telangiectasia

List Continues

ATAXIA* (*Continued*)

    E. Strümpell-Lorrain disease
    F. Cerebellar degeneration of Holmes
    G. Cerebellar atrophy of Marie-Foix-Alajouanine
    H. Azorean-Joseph-Machado disease
VII. Paraneoplastic
    a. Paraneoplastic subacute cerebellar degeneration
    B. Opsoclonus-myoclonus
VIII. Inherited neurometabolic disorder
    A. Wilson's disease
    B. Metachromatic leukodystrophy
    C. Lafora body disease
    D. Abetalipoproteinemia (Bassen-Kornzweig disease)
    E. Glutamate dehydrogenase deficiency
    F. Hereditary sensorimotor neuropathy type IV (Refsum's disease)
    G. Subacute necrotizing encephalomyelopathy (Leigh's disease)
    H. Adult neuronal ceroid-lipofuscinosis (Kufs disease)
    I. GM_2 gangliosidosis
    J. Cerebrotendinous xanthomatosis
    K. Amino/organic acid disorders
        1. Phenylketonuria
        2. Maple syrup urine disease
        3. Hartnup's disease
        4. Hyperalaninemia
    L. Urea cycle disorders
        1. Type II hyperammonemia
        2. Citrullinemia
        3. Argininosuccinic aciduria
        4. Hyperornithinemia

* Any sensory neuropathy with prominent loss of joint position sense can display prominent features of ataxia (see neuropathy list).

AKINETIC-RIGID SYNDROMES (PARKINSONISM)

I. Vascular
   A. Multi-infarct
   B. Binswanger's disease
   C. Amyloid angiopathy
II. Structural
   A. Mass lesions: subdural, AVM, tumor
   B. Normal pressure hydrocephalus
   C. Obstructive hydrocephalus
III. Metabolic
   A. Hypoparathyroidism with basal ganglia calcification
   B. Hepatocerebral degeneration
   C. Drugs and toxins
      1. Neuroleptics, dopamine receptor blockers, dopamine depletors
      2. Alpha-methyldopa
      3. Ethanol
      4. Lithium
      5. Carbon monoxide poisoning
      6. Carbon disulfide poisoning
      7. Manganese poisoning
      8. Mercury poisoning
      9. Methanol poisoning
      10. MPTP
      11. Cyanide poisoning
VI. Infectious
   A. Creutzfeldt-Jakob disease
   B. Encephalitis lethargica
   C. Neurosyphilis
   D. Other viral encephalitis
V. Neurodegenerative
   A. Parkinson's disease (idiopathic)
   B. Alzheimer's disease
   C. Olivopontocerebellar atrophy
   D. Shy-Drager syndrome
   E. Progressive supranuclear palsy
   F. Huntington's disease
   G. Azorean disease
   H. Striatonigral degeneration
   I. Corticobasal ganglionic degeneration
   J. Parkinson-ALS-dementia complex of Guam

List Continues

AKINETIC-RIGID SYNDROMES (PARKINSONISM)
(*Continued*)

    K. Pick's disease
    L. Corticostriatospinal degeneration ("spastic pseudosclerosis")
    M. Fahr's familial idiopathic basal ganglia calcification
    N. Pallidal degenerations
    O. Neuroacanthocytosis
    P. Dystonia-parkinsonism, L-dopa responsive
    Q. Chédiak-Higashi syndrome
  VI. Inherited neurometabolic disorder
    A. Wilson's disease
    B. Hallervorden-Spatz disease
    C. GM_1 gangliosidosis
    D. Gaucher's disease
 VII. Trauma
    A. "Punch-drunk syndrome"

(Modified from Weiner WJ, Lang AE: Movement Disorders: A Comprehensive Survey. Futura Publishing, Mount Kisco, New York, 1989, with permission.)

GAIT DISTURBANCES

Gait	Characteristics	Seen in
Ataxic (sensory)	Jerky, broad-based, slapping; worse with eyes closed.	Subacute combined degeneration, multiple sclerosis, tabes, sensory neuropathy.
Ataxic (cerebellar)	Wide-based, staggering, lurching; unable to walk tandem.	Lesions of vermis or cerebellar hemisphere (falls to same side as lesion).
Spastic	Arm held in flexion and adduction; leg(s) stiff, held in extension at hip and knee, plantar flexion of foot and toes; leg(s) circumducts; scissors gait in bilateral disease.	Lesion of one or both pyramidal pathways.
Parkinsonian	Slow, rigid, shuffling, small steps, stooped posture, propulsion (tendency to fall forward), festination (increase speed when walking), loss of associated movements (e.g., arm swing).	Various akinetic-rigid syndromes (see separate classification).
Marche à petits pas	Slow, short steps, shuffling, resembles parkinsonian gait.	Variety of cerebral or spinal disturbances.
Apraxia of gait	Slow, short steps, shuffling, but with normal tone, power, and sensation.	Frontal lobe lesions.
Steppage	Foot drop; foot drags, lifts high to avoid scraping floor.	Weakness of foot extensors: common/deep peroneal nerve, L4–L5, cauda equina lesions, or others.
Dystrophic (myopathic)	Lordosis, pelvis waddles and rotates, broad base.	Muscular dystrophy or other proximal myopathies.
Astasia-abasia	Bizarre, nondescript.	Hysterical.
Choreatic	Stuttering, dancing gait due to intermittent lordotic and flexion posturing.	Huntington's disease and other choreas.

FALLS IN THE ELDERLY

  I. Accident
 II. Senile (essential) gait disorder
III. Normal pressure hydocephalus
IV. Cervical spondylosis
 V. Lumbar stenosis
VI. Multisystem stability disorders
   A. Sensory
      1. Visual
         a. Decreased acuity
         b. Decreased dark adaptation
         c. Occular diseases
         d. Macular degeneration
         e. Glaucoma
         f. Cataracts
      2. Hearing impairment
         (May help orient and localize the person in space, especially
         with impairment of other sensory systems)
      3. Vestibular
         a. Age-related decline in function
         b. Vestibular degeneration
         c. Toxin
            (1) Aminoglycosides
            (2) Aspirin
            (3) Furosemide
            (4) Quinine
            (5) Quinidine
         d. Head trauma
         e. Otic surgery
         f. Middle ear infection
         g. Menière's disease
         h. Proprioceptive
   B. Peripheral neuropathy
      1. Low vitamin B_{12} especially common
   C. Posterior column (spine) disease
   D. Loss of cervical mechanoreceptors (e.g., after whiplash injury)
   E. Dementia
   F. Musculoskeletal
      1. Muscle
      2. Joints
      3. Bones

FALLS IN THE ELDERLY (*Continued*)

    4. Foot disorders
       a. Calluses
       b. Bunions
       c. Toe deformities
       d. Poor footwear
  G. Systemic diseases
     1. Decreased cerebral blood flow
     2. Cardiac arrhythmia
     3. Congestive heart failure
     4. Fatigue
     5. Confusion
     6. Shortness of breath
     7. Metabolic
     8. Electrolytes
     9. Hypothyroidism
    10. Acid-base disorders
  H. Postural hypotension
     1. Primary
     2. Volume depletion
     3. Decreased venous return from lower extremities
     4. Autonomic dysfunction
     5. Parkinson's disease
     6. Diabetes
     7. Age-related physiological changes
     8. Decreased functioning of the renin-angiotensin system
     9. Decreased baroreceptor sensitivity/carotid sinus hypersensitivity
    10. Drugs
  I. Medications
     1. Hypnotics
     2. Tranquilizers
     3. Antidepressants
     4. Antiarrhythmics
     5. Anticonvulsants
     6. Diuretics

(From Tinetti ME: Instability and falling in the elderly. Semin Neurol 9:39–45, 1989, with permission.)

SYNCOPE

I. Hypotension
    A. Vasomotor instability
        1. Vasovagal syncope
        2. Orthostatic hypotension
        3. Carotid sinus syndrome
        4. Micturition, defecation, cough, or swallow syncope
    B. Volume depletion
    C. Drugs (e.g., prazosin, nitrates)
II. Abnormal blood composition
    A. Hypoxemia
    B. Hypoglycemia
III. Cardiac disease
    A. Anatomic
        1. Aortic stenosis
        2. Mitral prolapse and regurgitation
        3. Hypertrophic cardiomyopathy
        4. Myxoma
        5. Pericardial tamponade
    B. Myocardial
        1. Ischemia and infarct
        2. Cardiomyopathy
        3. Pulmonary embolism
    C. Electrical
        1. Tachyarrhythmia
        2. Bradyarrhythmia
        3. Heart block (including drugs: e.g., quinidine)
        4. Sick sinus syndrome
        5. Carotid sinus sensitivity

SYNCOPE (*Continued*)

IV. Cerebral disorders
   A. Vascular insufficiency
   B. Seizures
 V. Psychiatric
   A. Hysterical
   B. Malingering
   C. Hyperventilation
VI. Metabolic
   A. Hypoglycemia
   B. Hypoxemia
VII. Miscellaneous
   A. Subclavian steal syndrome
   B. Takayasu's arteritis
   C. Glossopharyngeal neuralgia
   D. Pulmonary embolism

(From Lipsitz LA: Syncope in the elderly. Ann Intern Med 99:92–105, 1983, with permission.)

ORTHOSTATIC HYPOTENSION—COMMON CAUSES

I. Common
  A. Medications/toxins
    1. Alcohol
    2. Phenothiazines
    3. Calcium channel blockers
    4. Nitrates
    5. Diuretics
    6. Narcotics
    7. Sedatives
    8. Antiadrenergic medications
    9. Anticholinergic medications
    10. L-dopa
    11. Tricyclic antidepressants
    12. Lithium
    13. MAO inhibitors
    14. Neuroleptics
    15. Phenobarbital
    16. Vincristine
    17. Quinidine
  B. Dehydration
  C. Blood loss/anemia
  D. Hypokalemia
  E. Bedrest/deconditioning
  F. Malnutrition
II. Neurologic
  A. Central
    1. Stroke
    2. Tumors
    3. Parkinson's disease
    4. Shy-Drager syndrome

ORTHOSTATIC HYPOTENSION—COMMON CAUSES
(*Continued*)

  5. Myelopathy
  6. ?Depression
  7. ?Dementia
B. Peripheral
  1. Neuropathy
    a. Diabetes
    b. Amyloidosis
    c. Tabes dorsalis
    d. Alcoholic and nutritional
    e. Guillain-Barré syndrome
  2. Sympathectomy
III. Cardiovascular
  A. Cardiac
    1. Congestive heart failure
    2. Hypertrophic cardiomyopathy
    3. Mitral valve prolapse
  B. Peripheral vascular
    1. Large varicose veins
IV. Endocrine
  A. Adrenal insufficiency
  B. Pheochromocytoma
  C. Hypoaldosteronism/renal salt wasting
  D. Diabetes insipidus
V. Less common
  A. Idiopathic orthostatic hypotension
  B. Multiple system atrophy (Shy-Drager syndrome)
  C. Tumor associated (carcinoid, bradykinin)
  D. Baroreceptor destruction (neck radiation, surgery)

(From Mader SL: Orthostatic hypotension. Med Clin North Am 73:1337–1349, 1989, with permission.)

HYPOTHERMIA

I. Environmental exposure
   A. Extreme cold
   B. Chronic mild cold in susceptible individuals
II. Systemic disease
   A. Cardiovascular collapse
   B. Pneumonia
   C. Sepsis
   D. Tuberculous meningitis
   E. Uremia
   F. Failure of heat-generating systems
      1. Muscle-wasting diseases
      2. Cirrhosis
      3. Hepatic failure
      4. Protein deficiency
III. Endocrine/metabolic disturbances
   A. Hypothyroidism
   B. Hypopituitarism
   C. Addison's disease
   D. Hypoglycemia, ketoacidosis
IV. Drugs/toxins
   A. Ethanol, other alcohols
   B. Sedative drug intoxication
   C. Dopamine blockers (e.g., neuroleptics)
   D. Vasodilators
   E. Magnesium sulfate
   F. Yohimbine and clonidine
   G. Organophosphate poisoning
   H. Water intoxication

HYPOTHERMIA (*Continued*)

V. Hypothalamic dysfunction
   A. Diencephalic lesions
   B. Wernicke's encephalopathy
   C. Poikilothermy in premature infants
   D. Elderly or parkinsonian subjects
   E. Autonomic "storms" ("hypothalamic seizures")
VI. Other neurological causes
   A. Hepatic encephalopathy
   B. Multiple sclerosis
   C. Syndrome of episodic hyperhidrosis and hypothermia with or without agenesis of the corpus callosum
   D. Increased intracranial pressure
   E. Severe head injury
   F. Spinal cord transection

(From LeWitt PA, Eisenstadt J: Hypothermia. Neurol Forum 1:2–7, 1990, with permission.)

FECAL INCONTINENCE

I. Neurological problems
   A. Dementia
   B. Stroke
   C. Sedation
   D. Spinal cord or cauda equina compression
   E. Tabes dorsalis
   F. Multiple sclerosis
   G. Peripheral neuropathy
   H. Autonomic neuropathy
   I. Shy-Drager neuropathy
   J. Diabetes mellitus
II. Pelvic problems
   A. Trauma
   B. Injury
   C. Surgery (including hemorrhoidectomy)
   D. Childbirth
   E. Perineal descent
   F. Rectal ischemia
III. Miscellaneous
   A. Idiopathic hypoparathyroidism
   B. Acute myocardial infarction
   C. Splenomegaly

(From Schiller LR: Faecal incontinence. Clin Gastroenterol 15:687–704, 1986, with permission.)

Neuromuscular Symptoms and Syndromes

WEAKNESS (Upper Versus Lower Motor Neuron)

Lower Motor Neuron	Upper Motor Neuron
Weakness	Weakness
Marked atrophy	Minimal atrophy (disuse)
Fasciculations	No fasciculations
Decreased reflexes	Increased reflexes
No clonus	Clonus
No Babinski response	Babinski response
Root or nerve pattern	Pyramidal pattern of weakness (most affected: lower face, fine movements, upper limb extensors weaker than flexors, lower limb flexors weaker than extensors)

NEUROPATHY

I. Vasculitis/connective tissue disease
   (Most common presentation is mononeuritis multiplex)
   A. Polyarteritis nodosa
   B. Lupus
   C. Rheumatoid disease
   D. Sjögren syndrome
   E. Scleroderma
II. Demyelinating
   (Slowed nerve conduction)
   A. Acquired
      1. Guillain-Barré syndrome
      2. Diphtheria
      3. Chronic inflammatory/relapsing demyelinating neuropathy
      4. Paraproteinemia
         a. Myeloma
         b. Waldenström's macroglobulinemia
         c. Cryoglobulinemia
         d. Benign monoclonal gammopathy
   B. Inherited neurometabolic diseases
      1. Metachromatic leukodystrophy
      2. Krabbe's globoid body leukodystrophy
      3. Adrenoleukodystrophy
      4. Adrenomyeloneuropathy
      5. Abetalipoproteinemia (Bassen-Kornzweig syndrome)
      6. Alphalipoprotein deficiency (Tangier disease)
      7. Cherry-red spot myoclonus syndrome (type I)
      8. Cockayne syndrome
   C. Hereditary demyelinating neuropathies (also classified under "hereditary neuropathy")
      1. Hereditary sensorimotor neuropathy type I (Charcot-Marie-Tooth disease)
      2. Hereditary sensorimotor neuropathy type III (Dejerine-Sottas syndrome)
      3. Hereditary sensorimotor neuropathy type IV (Refsum's disease)
      4. Hereditary predisposition to pressure palsies
III. Metabolic
   A. Endocrine

NEUROPATHY (*Continued*)

1. Diabetes: clinical patterns of diabetic neuropathy
   a. Distal symmetrical
   b. Mixed (most common)
   c. Predominantly sensory (small, large fiber)
   d. Predominantly motor
   e. Predominantly autonomic
   f. Proximal motor ("amyotrophy")
   g. Focal/multifocal neuropathy
   h. Mononeuritis multiplex
   i. Cranial neuropathy
   j. Intercostal neuropathy
   k. Entrapment neuropathies (e.g., carpal tunnel)
2. Hypothyroidism
3. Acromegaly
B. Drugs
   1. General: phenytoin, tricyclics, INH, hydralazine, nitrofurantoin, amiodarone, disulfiram, metronidazole, dapsone
   2. Antineoplastic: vincristine, Adriamycin, cisplatin
C. Toxins
   1. Alcohol
   2. Metals
   3. Arsenic
   4. Lead
   5. Mercury
   6. Thallium
   7. Industrial toxins
   8. *N*-hexane
   9. Acrylamide
   10. Methylbutyl ketone
   11. Triorthocresylphosphate
   12. Carbon disulfide
D. Nutritional
   1. Vitamin B_1 (thiamin) deficiency (Beriberi)
   2. Vitamin B_6 (pyridoxine) deficiency/excess
   3. Vitamin B_{12} (cobalamin) deficiency
   4. Pantothenic acid deficiency
   5. Nicotinic acid deficiency (pellagra)
   6. Folate deficiency
   7. Vitamin E deficiency

List Continues

NEUROPATHY (*Continued*)

   E. Porphyria
   F. Organ failure
      1. Uremia
      2. Hyperglycemia/hypoglycemia
      3. Hypophosphatemia
IV. Infectious
   A. Bacterial
      1. Leprosy
      2. Sarcoid
      3. Bacterial endocarditis
   B. Viral
      1. Hepatitis B
      2. Mononucleosis
      3. Herpes zoster
      4. HIV
   C. Spirochetes
      1. Lyme disease
   D. Tick paralysis
 V. Paraneoplastic
   A. Carcinoma (lung 50%)
   B. Lymphoma
   C. Leukemia
   D. Paraproteinemias (see above)
   E. Amyloid
      1. With primary (including myeloma-associated amyloid) and familial amyloid only
VI. Inherited
   A. Hereditary neuropathy
      1. Hereditary sensorimotor neuropathy (HSMN)
         a. HSMN type I (Charcot-Marie-Tooth disease)*
         b. HSMN type II (Charcot-Marie-Tooth/axonal type)*

NEUROPATHY (*Continued*)

      c. HSMN type III (Dejerine-Sottas syndrome)

      d. HSMN type IV (Refsum's disease)

      e. HSMN type V

      f. HSMN type VI

      g. HSMN type VII

   2. Hereditary predisposition to pressure palsies

   3. Hereditary sensory neuropathy (HSN)

      a. HSN type I

      b. HSN type II ("congenital sensory neuropathy")

      c. NSN type III (Riley-Day syndrome)

      d. HSN type IV ("congenital sensory neuropathy with anhidrosis")

      e. Congenital insensitivity to pain

  B. Inherited neurometabolic disorders

   1. Fabry's disease

   2. GM_2 gangliosidosis

   3. Inherited disorders resulting in demyelinating neuropathy (see above)

VII. Trauma

  A. Mechanical

  B. Radiation

  C. Cold

* Note that type I Charcot-Marie-Tooth disease is demyelinating, whereas type II is an axonal neuropathy.

TYPICAL CLINICAL DEFICITS SEEN WITH
PROXIMAL NERVE LESIONS

Nerve	Impairment
Musculocutaneous	Forearm flexion at elbow, supination
Radial	Forearm extension, flexion, supination Write extension Thumb extension, abduction in plane of palm
Median	Forearm pronation Wrist flexion Finger flexion (digits 2 and 3) Thumb flexion, opposition, abduction at right angle to palm
Ulnar	Wrist flexion, adduction Abduction and adduction of all digits Finger flexion (digits 4 and 5) Flex, rotate digit 5
Obturator	Thigh adduction
Femoral	Thigh flexion at hip Leg extension at knee
Sciatic	Leg flexion at knee
Tibial	Foot plantar flexion, inversion Toe flexion, cup sole
Superficial peroneal	Foot eversion
Deep peroneal	Foot dorsiflexion, toe extension

(From Devinsky O, Feldmann E: Anatomy. p. 1. In Examination of the Cranial and Peripheral Nerves. Churchill Livingstone, New York, 1988, with permission.)

MYOPATHY

I. Inflammatory myopathy
   A. Polymyositis/dermatomyositis
   B. Lupus
   C. Polyarteritis nodosa
   D. Rheumatoid disease
   E. Mixed connective tissue disease
   F. Scleroderma
   G. Sjögren syndrome
   H. Sarcoid
II. Acquired metabolic disorders
   A. Endocrine
      1. Steroids (Cushing's syndrome, iatrogenic)
      2. Hyperthyroidism
      3. Hypothyroidism
      4. Hyperparathyroidism
      5. Acromegaly
   B. Drugs/toxins
      1. Alcohol
      2. Chloroquine
      3. Colchicine
      4. Vincristine
   C. Organ failure
      1. Uremic neuromyopathy
III. Inherited metabolic disorders
   A. Glycogen storage
      1. Acid maltase deficiency (type II, Pompe's disease)
      2. Debrancher enzyme deficiency (type III)
      3. Myophosphorylase deficiency (type V, McArdle's disease)
      4. Phosphofructokinase deficiency (type VII, Tarui's disease)
   B. Lipid storage
      1. Carnitine deficiency
      2. Carnitine palmityltransferase deficiency
   C. Mitochondrial encephalomyopathy
      1. Kearns-Sayre syndrome
      2. MERRF (myoclonal epilepsy with red ragged fibers)
      3. MELAS (mitochondrial myopathy, encephalopathy, lactic acidosis, stroke-like episodes)
      4. Defects of the respiratory chain
         a. Complex I, III
         b. Complex IV (cytochrome c oxidase)

List Continues

MYOPATHY (*Continued*)

    c. Fatal infantile mitochondrial myopathy
    d. Benign infantile mitochondrial myopathy
    e. Trichopoliodystrophy (Menkes disease)
    f. Subacute necrotizing encephalomyelopathy (Leigh's disease)
    g. Progressive sclerosing poliodystrophy (Alpers syndrome)
  D. Miscellaneous
    1. Malignant hyperthermia
    2. Periodic paralysis
    3. Hypokalemic
    4. Hyperkalemic/normokalemic periodic paralysis
    5. Hyperthyroidism with hypokalemic paralysis
    6. Paramyotaonia congenita (Eulenburg's disease)
IV. Degenerative muscular dystrophy
  A. Pseudohypertrophic
    1. Duchenne type
    2. Becker type
  B. Facioscapulohumeral dystrophy
  C. Limb-girdle dystrophy.
  D. Myotonic dystrophy
  E. Oculopharyngeal
  F. Distal myopathy
  G. Emery-Dreifuss dystrophy
  H. Scapuloperoneal dystrophy
V. Congenital myopathy
  A. Nemaline
  B. Centronuclear (myotubular)
  C. Central core
  D. Congenital fiber type disproportion
VI. Paraneoplastic myopathy
  A. Polymyositis/dermatomyositis
VII. Infectious/postinfectious myopathy
  A. Viral myositis (e.g., influenza, adenovirus)
  V. Inclusion body myositis
  C. Cysticercosis
  D. Trichinosis
  E. HIV
  F. Toxoplasmosis

MUSCLE CRAMPS—ASSOCIATED CONDITIONS

I. True cramp (motor unit hyperactivity)
  A. Ordinary cramp (overwork, exercise, charley horse)
  B. Lower motor neuron disease
      1. Amyotrophic lateral sclerosis
      2. Motor neuropathies
      3. Peripheral nerve injuries
      4. Root compression
      5. Old polio
  C. Hemodialysis/uremia
  D. Heat cramp
  E. Fluid and electrolyte disorders
      1. Hypoglycemia
      2. Salt depletion (perspiration, diarrhea, vomiting, diuretics)
  F. Drug-induced cramp
      1. Nifedipine
      2. Beta-agonists: terbutaline, salbutamol
      3. Alcohol
      4. Clofibrate
      5. Penicillamine
  G. Nocturnal leg cramps in the elderly
II. Contracture (electrically silent)
  A. Metabolic myopathy (e.g., McArdle's disease)
  B. Thyroid disease
III. Tetany (sensory and motor unit hyperactivity)
  A. Hypocalcemia
  B. Respiratory alkalosis
  C. Hypomagnesemia
  D. Hypokalemia, hyperkalemia

(From McGee SR: Muscle cramps. Arch Intern Med 150:511–518, 1990, with permission.)

MYOTONIA

    I. Hyperkalemic/normokalemic periodic paralysis
   II. Myotonic dystrophy
  III. Myotonia congenita of Thomsen
  IV. Hypothyroidism (pseudomyotonia)
   V. Myotonic chondrodystrophy (Schwartz-Jampel syndrome)
  VI. Diazocholesterol
 VII. Aromatic amino acids
VIII. Clofibrate
  IX. Paramyotonia congenita (Eulenburg's disease)
   X. Isaacs syndrome
  XI. Acid maltase deficiency (type II, Pompe's disease)

MYALGIA*

I. Direct trauma
II. Ischemia
III. Muscle use/overuse
    A. Occupational
IV. Nocturnal/resting
V. Idiopathic in children
VI. Inflammatory/immune
    A. Infection (viral, bacterial, fungal, parasitic)
    B. Idiopathic
        1. Dermatomyositis/polymyositis
        2. Sarcoidosis (nodular)
        3. Eosinophilic myositis
        4. Focal nodular myositis
    C. Connective tissue disorders
        1. Rheumatoid arthritis
        2. Progressive systemic sclerosis
        3. Systemic lupus erythematosus
        4. Vasculitis
        5. Sjögren syndrome
        6. Polymyalgia rheumatica
    D. Primary fibromyalgia
    E. Chronic myalgia/fatigue
        1. Postviral
    F. Thrombophlebitis
VII. Metabolic
    A. Enzyme defects
        1. Myophosphorylase deficiency (McArdle's disease)
        2. Carnitine palmityl transferase (CPT) deficiency
        3. Myoadenylate deaminase (MADA) deficiency
        4. NADH-coenzyme Q reductase (complex I) deficiency
    B. Endocrine
        1. Hypothyroidism
        2. Hypoadrenalism
        3. Hypoparathyroidism
    C. Mineral/electrolyte
        1. Hypokalemia
        2. Hypocalcemia
        3. Hypomagnesemia
        4. Hypophosphatemia
        5. Hyponatremia
    D. Other

List Continues

MYALGIA* (*Continued*)

    1. Pregnancy
    2. Liver cirrhosis
    3. Uremia
    4. Hemodialysis
    5. Severe malnutrition
VIII. Drug/toxin
    A. Alcohol
    B. Clofibrate
    C. Epsilon-aminocaproic acid
    D. Heroin
    E. Amphetamine
    F. Phencyclidine
    G. Vincristine
    H. Cimetidine
    I. Lithium
    J. Trazodone
    K. Related to hypokalemia (diuretics, glycyrrhizinic acid, carbenoxolone, amphotericin B)
    L. Animal venom (snake and spider)
    M. Tetanus toxoid
    N. Strychnine
    O. Penicillamine
  IX. Neurological
    A. Myopathy
      1. Becker type, myotonia congenita
    B. Neuropathy
      1. Brachial neuritis, chronic inflammatory polyneuropathy, acute intermittent porphyria, diabetic amyotrophy
    C. Motor neuron
      1. Amyotrophic lateral sclerosis, poliomyelitis
    D. CNS
      1. Parkinson's disease
      2. Multiple sclerosis
      3. "Stiff man" syndrome
  X. Psychiatric

* Myalgia is any discomfort in the muscle. A cramp is a sudden, involuntary, and painful muscle contraction. All cramps can be considered as causes of myalgia, but the converse is not true.
(From Roy EP, Gutman L: Myalgia. Neurol Clin 6:621–636, 1988, with permission.)

Headache and Facial Pain

HEADACHE

I. Muscle contraction
   A. Tension/stress
   B. Mixed tension/vascular
   C. Eyestrain
   D. Cervical spondylosis or other cervical spine pathology
   E. Post-traumatic
II. Vascular headache
   A. Common migraine
   B. Classic migraine
   C. Atypical migraine
   D. Perimenstrual headache
   E. Underlying metabolic cause
      1. Fever
      2. Hypoxia
      3. Hypoglycemia
      4. Drugs/toxins
         a. Alcohol
         b. Nitrates/nitrites
         c. Hydralazine
         d. Carbon monoxide poisoning
         e. Benzene
         f. Carbon tetrachloride
         g. Lead poisoning
         h. Arsenic poisoning
         i. Carbon disulphide poisoning
      5. Pheochromocytoma
   F. Cluster headaches
      1. Typical cluster
      2. Chronic cluster
      3. Paroxysmal hemicrania
   G. Underlying vascular disease
      1. Hypertension
      2. Ischemic stroke (especially embolic)
      3. Dissection
III. Inflammation/meningeal irritation/traction
   A. Secondary to sinus/ocular/ear disease
   B. Parenchymal hemorrhage
   C. Subarachnoid hemorrhage
   D. AVM

List Continues

HEADACHE (*Continued*)

    E. Chronic subdural
    F. Meningitis
    G. Pseudotumor cerebri
    H. Brain tumors
    I. Abscess
    J. CNS vasculitis (see separate classification)
    K. Giant cell (temporal) arteritis
    L. Lumbar puncture headache
IV. Miscellaneous
    A. Glaucoma
    B. Temporomandibular joint disease
    C. Dental disease
    D. Exercise
    E. Coughing/straining
    F. Coital headache
 V. Psychogenic/malingering

CHARACTERISTICS OF MIGRAINOUS AND TENSION HEADACHES

	Migraine (%)	Tension (%)
Age of onset		
<20 yr	55	30
>20 yr	45	70
Premonitory symptoms	60	10
Frequency		
Daily	3	50
<Weekly	60	15
Constant, daily	0	20
Duration		
1–3 d	35	10
Throbbing pain	80	30
Location of pain		
Unilateral	80	10
Bilateral	20	90
Vomiting with attacks	50	10
Family history of headache	65	40

(From Raskin NH: Tension headache. p. 215. In Headache. Churchill Livingstone, New York, 1988, with permission.)

SYMPTOMS ACCOMPANYING MIGRAINE HEADACHE

Symptom	Percent Affected
Nausea	87
Vomiting	56
Diarrhea	16
Photophobia	82
Visual disturbances	36
Fortification spectra	10
Photopsia	26
Paresthesia	33
Scalp tenderness	65
Lightheadedness	72
Vertigo	33
Alteration in consciousness	18
Seizure	4
Syncope	10
Confusional state	4

(From Raskin NH: Migraine: clinical aspects. p. 35. In Headache. Churchill Livingstone, New York, 1988, with permission.)

FACTORS PRECIPITATING MIGRAINE ATTACKS

Common Factors	Less Common Factors
Stress and worry	High humidity
Menstruation	Excessive sleep
Oral contraceptives	High-altitude exposure
Glare, dazzle	Excessive vitamin A
Physical exertion, fatigue	Drugs: nitroglycerine, histamine,
Lack of sleep	reserpine, hydralazine, estrogen,
Hunger	corticosteroid withdrawal
Head trauma	Cold foods
Food and beverages containing	Reading
nitrate, glutamate, salt, aspartame,	Refractive errors
tyramine, and other, as yet	Pungent odors: perfumes, organic
unidentified, chemicals (most	solvents, smoke
common foods: chocolate, wine,	Fluorescent lighting
dairy products, citrus fruits, beer,	Allergic reactions
fried/fatty foods, pork, onions, tea,	
coffee, seafood)	
Weather or ambient temperature	
changes	
Lack of sleep	

(From Raskin NH: Migraine: clinical aspects. p. 35. In Headache. Churchill Livingstone, New York, 1988, with permission.)

MAJOR CRITERIA FOR THE DIAGNOSIS OF LATE-LIFE MIGRAINE ACCOMPANIMENTS*

   I. Fortification spectrum or other visual hallucinations in the attack
  II. Slow evolution of visual and sensory symptoms
 III. Serial progression with delays from one accompaniment to another
  IV. Two or more identical attacks (weighs against embolism)
   V. Duration greater than 20 minutes (weighs against TIA)
  VI. Midlife flurry of attacks
 VII. Complete recovery from attacks
VIII. Normal angiography (weighs against thrombosis)
  IX. Exclusion of the following:
      A. Cerebral thrombosis
      B. Embolism
      C. Dissection
      D. Epilepsy
      E. Thrombocytopenia
      F. Polycythemia
      G. Thrombotic thrombocytopenia
      H. Hyperviscosity syndromes
      I. Lupus anticoagulant

* The major purpose of recognizing this disorder is to distinguish it from TIAs. The treatment and prognosis for these disorders are different.
(From Raskin NH: Migraine: clinical aspects. p. 35. In Headache. Churchill Livingstone, 1988, with permission.)

SYMPTOMS THAT MAY REPRESENT MIGRAINE EQUIVALENTS

I. Visual
  A. Photopsia (flashes of light)
  B. Scotomata (island of impaired vision)
  C. Hemianopia
  D. Diplopia
  E. Blindness
  F. Metamorphopsia (objects appearing misshapen)
II. Neurological
  A. Amnesia
  B. Confusion or coma
  C. Hemiparesis
  D. Paresthesia
  E. Vertigo
  F. Hearing loss
  G. Episodic mood changes
III. Other
  A. Abdominal pain
  B. Cyclic vomiting
  C. Coronary artery spasm
  D. Episodic fever

(From Kunke RS: Migraine aura without headache. Pain Management 3:176–182, 1990, with permission.)

PREVENTIVE THERAPY FOR MIGRAINE HEADACHE

Drug	Tablet Size (mg)	Daily Dose Range (mg)	Most Common Side Effects
Ergonovine	0.2	0.4–2.0	Nausea, abdominal pain, leg "tiredness"
Amitriptyline	10, 25, 50, 75, 100	10–175	Sedation, dry mouth, weight gain
Propranolol	10, 20, 40, 60, 80, 90; sustained release: 60, 80, 120, 160	40–320	Lethargy, insomnia, constipation, lightheadedness
Papaverine	150, 300	300–900	Nausea
Cyproheptadine	4	12–32	Sedation, weight gain
Ergotamine, phenobarbital, belladona (Cafergot P-B)		1–4 tablets	Nausea, sedation
Phenelzine	15	15–75	Insomnia, lightheadedness, constipation, orthostatic hypotension
Methysergide	2	2–8	Nausea, abdominal pain, muscle cramps, insomnia, weight gain, edema, peripheral vasoconstriction; retroperitoneal, pleuropulmonary, and cardiac fibrosis infrequent but important
Naproxen	250, 275, 375, 500	1,000–1,650	Nausea, abdominal pain, fluid retention
Verapamil	80, 120; sustained release: 240	160–480	Constipation, lightheadedness, nausea, fluid retention, hypotension
Flunarizine	5, 10	5–15	Sedation, weight gain

(From Raskin NH: Migraine: treatment. p. 156. In Headache. Churchill Livingstone, New York, 1988, with permission.)

CLINICAL FEATURES OF GIANT CELL ARTERITIS

Incidence of Common Features at Initial Evaluation	Percentage
Headache	85
Temporal artery tenderness	70
Jaw claudication	65
Lingual, limb, or swallowing claudication	20
Brachiocephalic bruits	50
Thickened or nodular temporal artery	45
Pulseless temporal artery	40
Visual symptoms	40
Fixed blindness, partial or complete	15
Polymyalgia rheumatica	40
Weight loss >6 kg	35
ESR > 50 mm/hr	95
ESR > 100 mm/hr	60
Fever (>37.5°C)	20
Abnormal liver function	50
Anemia (Hct < 35%)	50

Less Common, but Characteristic Features

Raynaud's phenomenon of limbs or tongue
Tender scalp nodules
Thick, tender occipital arteries
Necrotic lesions of scalp, tongue
Carotid artery tenderness
Swelling of the hands
Taste, smell disturbances
Distended, beaded retinal vessels
Diminished or absent radial artery pulses
Mononeuropathy: median, peroneal, cervical root

(From Raskin NH: Giant cell arteritis. p. 317. In Headache. Churchill Livingstone, New York, 1988, with permission.)

CLUSTER HEADACHE

I. Clinical stereotype
  A. Disorder of men
  B. Peak age of onset 20–50 years
  C. Paroxysmal, explosive, unilateral, periorbital pain
  D. "Clock" mechanism, often nocturnal (i.e., occurs at same time each night)
  E. Cluster cycles (lasting weeks)
  F. Pain-free intervals (lasting months)
  G. Ipsilateral nasal stuffiness, soft tissue swelling, forehead swelling, lacrimation, hyperemic eye, Horner syndrome
  H. Alcohol sensitivity during cluster cycles

Frequency of most commonly associated symptoms	Incidence (%)
Lacrimation	84
Conjunctival injection	58
Ptosis	57
Blocked nostril	48
Rhinorrhea	43
Bradycardia	43
Nausea	40
General perspiration	26

(From Raskin NH: Cluster headache. p. 229. In Headache. Churchill Livingstone, New York, 1988, with permission.)

CHARACTERISTIC OF CRANIAL NEURALGIAS

I. Trigeminal neuralgia
   A. Electric shock-like, machine gun-like pain volleys
   B. Presence of trigger maneuvers
   C. Unilateral pain: V_2, V_3 most commonly
   D. Rarely nocturnal
   E. Absence of neurological deficit
   F. Refractory periods
   G. Dramatic abatement with intravenous phenytoin
II. Glossopharyngeal neuralgia
   A. One-minute "square wave" paroxysms
   B. Submandibular or aural pain
   C. Taste, cold, swallowed stimuli are common triggers
   D. Prominent cluster tempo
   E. Nocturnal attacks common
   F. Refractory periods
   G. Coexists with trigeminal neuralgia
   H. Dramatically ceases after intravenous phenytoin

(Modified from Raskin NH: Facial pain. p. 333. In Headache. Churchill Livingstone, New York, 1988, with permission.)

5
EMERGENCY NEUROLOGY

COMA AND CONFUSION

I. Without focal signs, without meningismus
  A. Metabolic
    1. Anoxia/hypoperfusion
    2. Hyperglycemia
    3. Hypoglycemia
    4. Hypercalcemia
    5. Deranged ionic environment
      a. Sodium
      b. Acidosis/alkalosis
      c. Magnesium
    6. Inadequate supply of other substrates
      a. Thiamine deficiency (acute Wernicke's disease)
      b. Hypothyroidism
      c. Addison's disease
      d. Vitamin B_{12} deficiency (mostly confusion, dementia)
  B. Toxic
    1. Endogenous
      a. Sepsis
      b. Uremia
      c. Hepatic encephalopathy
      d. Ketoacidosis
      e. Hypercarbia
      f. Reye syndrome
      g. Porphyria
      h. Urea cycle disorders
    2. Exogenous
      a. Alcohol
      b. Opiates
      c. Barbiturates
      d. Anticholinergics (e.g., tricyclics)
      e. Neuroleptics
      f. Carbon monoxide poisoning
      g. Cyanide poisoning
  C. Seizures: ictal/postictal
  D. Infection: encephalitis
  E. Hypertensive encephalopathy
  F. Concussion: usually no focal signs

List Continues

COMA AND CONFUSION (*Continued*)

II. Without focal signs, but with meningismus
   A. Infection
      1. Bacterial meningitis
      2. Viral meningoencephalitis
      3. Fungal meningitis
   B. Subarachnoid hemorrhage
III. With focal signs
   A. Vascular
      1. Infarction
         a. Thrombotic
         b. Embolic
         c. Vasculitis
         d. Vasospasm (e.g., postsubarachnoid hemorrhage)
         e. Dissection
         f. Venous thrombosis
   B. Structural
      1. Hemorrhage
         a. Hypertensive
         b. Aneurysm
         c. Bleeding diathesis (leukemia, anticoagulants)
         d. Amyloid angiopathy
      2. Subdural/epidural hematoma
      3. Tumor (primary or secondary, with or without hemorrhage or increased intracranial pressure)
      4. AVM
   C. Infection
      1. Bacterial (cerebritis, abscess, TB)
      2. Viral
      3. Fungal
      4. Parasitic
   D. Trauma

GLASGOW COMA SCALE

Best motor response	
Obeys	6
Localizes pain	5
Withdraws	4
Flexion to pain	3
Extension to pain	2
Nil	1
Best verbal response	
Oriented	5
Confused conversation	4
Inappropriate words	3
Incomprehensible sounds	2
Nil	1
Eye opening	
Spontaneously	4
To speech	3
To pain	2
Nil	1

(From Jennett B, Teasdale G: Aspects of coma after severe head injury. Lancet 1:878–881, 1977, with permission.)

EMERGENCY MANAGEMENT OF COMA

    I. Assure clear airway and oxygenation: intubation, tracheostomy, blood gases
    II. Maintain systemic circulation: administer IV fluids, hypertensive/hypotensive agents to maintain mean arterial pressure at approximately 100 mmHg (higher in known hypertensive patients or with increased intracranial pressure)
    III. Give 50–100 mg thiamine parenterally
    IV. Draw blood for chemistry and toxicology (see separate list), then give 25 g glucose (50 ml of 50% solution)
    V. Lower intracranial pressure (see separate list)
    VI. Stop seizures (see separate list)
    VII. Treat infection: blood cultures, LP if indicated; then administer antibiotics
    VIII. Restore acid base, electrolyte balance
    IX. Adjust body temperature by heating or cooling as necessary
    X. Consider specific antidotes (see separate list)
    XI. Control agitation with minor or major tranquilizers when the diagnosis is relatively clear and therapy is directed at underlying cause
    XII. Protect the eyes from exposure keratitis by lubrication with ophthalmic ointment and passive closing with tape or corneal bandage

(From Plum F, Posner JB: Approach to the unconscious patient. pp. 347–350. In The Diagnosis of Stupor and Coma, 3rd Ed. FA Davis, Philadelphia, 1980, with permission.)

EMERGENCY LABORATORY TESTS FOR
METABOLIC COMA

I. Immediate tests
  A. Venous blood
    1. Glucose
    2. Electrolytes (Na, K, Cl, CO_2, Ca, PO_4)
    3. Urea or creatinine
    4. Osmolality
  B. Arterial blood
    1. Check color
    2. pH
    3. PO_2
    4. PCO_2
    5. HCO_3
    6. Carboxyhemoglobin
  C. CSF
    1. Cells
    2. Gram stain
    3. Glucose
  D. EKG
II. Deferred tests
  A. Venous blood
    1. Sedative and toxic drugs
    2. Liver function
    3. Coagulation studies
    4. Thyroid function
    5. Adrenal function
    6. Blood cultures
    7. Viral titers
  B. Urine
    1. Sedative and toxic drugs
    2. Culture
  C. CSF
    1. Protein
    2. Culture
    3. Viral and fungal titers

(From Plum F, Posner JB: Approach to the unconscious patient. p. 358. In The Diagnosis of Stupor and Coma, 3rd Ed. FA Davis, Philadelphia, 1980, with permission.)

BREATHING PATTERNS AND ASSOCIATED CNS LEVEL

Respiratory Pattern	Characteristics	Site of Lesion
Cheyne-Stokes respiration	Phases of hyperpnea regularly alternating with apnea	Forebrain
Central neurogenic hyperventilation	Sustained, rapid, and deep hyperpnea	Low midbrain, upper pontine tegmentum
Apneustic respiration	Prolonged inspiration followed by a pause of 2–3 s before expiration	Mid or caudal pons
Cluster breathing	Groups of breaths (clusters) separated by apnea	Mid or rostral pons
Ataxic respiration (Biot's respiration)	Completely irregular pattern	Medulla

HERNIATION SYNDROMES

Uncal Herniation
The uncus, the medial part of the temporal lobe, is pushed medially and through the tentorial notch, compressing structures in and near the midbrain.

Structures	Clinical Manifestation
CN III (ipsilateral)	Third nerve palsy (ocular paresis, large pupil)
Posterior cerebral artery	Occipital infarction (homonymous hemianopsia)
Midbrain (including cerebral peduncles)	Obtundation
	Hemiparesis (80% ipsilateral, 20% contralateral)
	Late → decorticate posturing → decerebrate posturing

Central Herniation
Often seen with more medial or global swelling, the hemispheres and midbrain are compressed more symmetrically.

Structures	Clinical Manifestation
Diencephalon	Decreased consciousness
	Small pupils (reactive)
	Cheyne-Stokes respiration
Midbrain/pons	Coma
	Midposition pupils (fixed)
	Hemi- or quadriparesis → decorticate posturing
	Abnormal breathing (central hyperventilation, apneustic breathing)
Pons/medulla (late)	Coma
	Decerebrate posturing
	Apneustic breathing, cluster breathing
	Apnea
	Cushing response (slowed pulse, increased blood pressure)
	Death

List Continues

HERNIATION SYNDROMES (*Continued*)

Tonsilar Herniation
Increased pressure in the posterior fossa pushes the cerebellar tonsils downward through the foramen magnum.

Structures	**Clinical Manifestation**
Medulla	Coma
	Stiff neck
	Vomiting
	Skew deviation of the eyes
	Irregular breathing (ataxic)
	Apnea
	Death

Upward Herniation
Posterior fossa mass pushes upper brainstem and cerebellum through the tentorial opening.

Structures	**Clinical Manifestation**
Midbrain/pons	Coma
	Small pupils (reactive early in compression)
	Abnormal occulocephalics and caloric responses (especially loss of vertical eye movements)
	Abnormal breathing (central hyperventillation, apneustic breathing)
	Hemi- or quadriparesis → decorticate posturing

TREATMENT OF INCREASED INTRACRANIAL PRESSURE

I. Elevate head, facing forward (to prevent jugular compression)
II. Hyperventilation: intubate and decrease PCO_2 to 20–25 mmHg
III. Hyperosmolar agents: mannitol 25% solution, 1.5–2 g/kg bolus injection
IV. Steroids if appropriate (16–100 mg dexamethasone daily): decreases edema around certain lesions such as brain tumors and sub- and epidural hematomas, improve brain compliance, diminishes plateau waves (may also add diuretics such as furosemide or acetazolamide)
V. Insert Foley catheter and measure urine output
VI. Avoid patient agitation
VII. Monitor osmolality and electrolytes frequently
VIII. ?Barbiturate anesthesia for traumatic coma
IX. Definitive treatment aimed at underlying lesion

CLINICAL FEATURES OF CEREBELLAR
HEMORRHAGE AND INFARCT*

Symptoms	Signs
Early stage	
Headache	Truncal ataxia
Dizziness	Nystagmus
Nausea	Appendicular ataxia
Vomiting	Stiff neck
Lack of balance	Dysarthria
Intermediate stage	
Irritability	Pseudo-VI palsy
Confusion	VI palsy
Drowsiness	Gaze paresis
	Forced gaze deviation
	Babinski signs
	Peripheral facial palsy
	Horner syndrome
	Mild hemiparesis
	Small pupils reactive to bright light
Late stage	
Stupor	Pinpoint pupils
Coma	Ataxic respirations
Posturing	Apnea
Cardiovascular instability	

* The clinical syndrome of cerebellar hemorrhage is reviewed in detail because of the great importance of early recognition of this syndrome. It is one of the true neurological emergencies.

(From Heros RC: Cerebellar hemorrhage and infarction. Stroke 13:106–109, 1982, with permission.)

MANAGEMENT OF GENERALIZED TONIC-CLONIC STATUS EPILEPTICUS

Time From Start of Therapy	Procedure
0 min	Assess cardiorespiratory function as the presence of tonic-clonic status is confirmed. If unsure of diagnosis, observe one tonic-clonic attack and verify the presence of unconsciousness after the end of the tonic-clonic attack. Insert oral airway and administer O_2. Insert IV line. Draw venous blood for CBC, electrolytes, glucose, urea, calcium, magnesium, and anticonvulsant levels. Draw arterial blood for immediate determination of pH, PO_2, PCO_2, HCO_3. Monitor respiration, blood pressure, and EKG (and EEG if possible).
5 min	Start IV infusion of normal saline containing vitamin B complex. Give bolus injection of 50 ml 50% glucose.
10 min	Infuse diazepam IV no faster than 2 mg/min until seizures stop or until a total of 20 mg, *or* infuse lorazepam 4 mg IV over 1 min (repeat once in 10 min). Also start infusion of phenytoin no faster than 50 mg/min to a total of 18 mg/kg. If hypotension develops, slow infusion rate. (Phenytoin 50 mg/ml in propylene glycol may be placed in a 100-ml volume-control set and diluted with normal saline. Watch infusion rate very carefully. Alternatively, phenytoin may be administered by slow IV push).
30–40 min	If seizures persist, two options are available: IV phenobarbital or diazepam drip. The two drugs should not be given in the same patient; an endotracheal tube should now be inserted.
	IV phenobarbital option: start infusion of phenobarbital no faster than 100 mg/min until seizures stop or to a loading dose of 20 mg/kg.
	or
	Diazepam IV drip option: 100 mg of diazepam is diluted in 500 ml 5% dextrose in water and run in at 40 ml/hr. This ensures diazepam serum levels of 0.2 to 0.8 μg/ml.
50–60 min	If seizures continue, general anesthesia with isoflurane is instituted. If an anesthesiologist is not immediately available, start infusion of 4% solution of paraldehyde in normal saline; administer at a rate fast enough to stop seizures, *or* 50–100 mg lidocaine may be given by IV push. If initial lidocaine bolus is ineffective, 50–100 mg diluted in 250 ml of 5% dextrose in water should be dripped IV at a rate of 1–2 mg/min.

List Continues

MANAGEMENT OF GENERALIZED TONIC-CLONIC
STATUS EPILEPTICUS (*Continued*)

Time From Start of Therapy	Procedure
80 min	If paraldehyde or lidocaine has not terminated seizures within 20 min from start of infusion, general anesthesia with halothane and neuromuscular junction blockade must be given. If status epilepticus reappears when general anesthesia is stopped, a neurologist who is an expert on status epilepticus should be consulted. Advice from a regional epilepsy center should also be sought on the management of intractable status.

(Modified from Delgado-Escueta AV, Wasterlain C, Treiman DM, Porter RJ: Management of status epilepticus. N Engl J Med 306:1337–1340, 1982, with permission.)

EMERGENCY ANTIDOTES

Toxin	Antidote
Acetaminophen	*N*-acetylcysteine
Arsenic	Dimercaprol (BAL)
Atropine, other anticholinegics	Physostigmine
Carbon monoxide	Oxygen
Cyanide	Amyl nitrite, sodium nitrite
Ethylene glycol	Ethanol
Lead	Calcium disodium versenate
Mercury	Dimercaprol (BAL)
Methanol	Ethanol
Opiates, propoxyphene	Naloxone
Organophosphates	Atropine, followed by pralidoxime chloride (2-PAM chloride)
Phenothiazines (acute dystonic reactions)	Diphenhydramine, benztropine mesylate

(From Schwartz JF: Poisonings and drug-induced neurological diseases. pp. 909–924. In Swaiman KF: Pediatric Neurology: Principles and Practice. CV Mosby, St. Louis, 1989, with permission.)

ACUTE RESPIRATORY FAILURE—
NEUROMUSCULAR CAUSES

  I. Spinal cord
   A. Trauma, upper cervical segments
   B. Tetanus
 II. Lower motor neuron
   A. Amyotrophic lateral sclerosis/motor neuron disease
   B. Poliomyelitis
   C. Rabies
III. Peripheral nerve
   A. Guillain-Barré syndrome
   B. Porphyria
   C. Hyperkalemic periodic paralysis
   D. Diphtheria
   E. Ciguatera toxin
   F. Saxitoxin
   G. Tetrodotoxin
   H. Thallium
   I. Buckthorn berry toxin
 IV. Neuromuscular junction
   A. Myasthenia gravis
   B. Botulism
   C. Hypermagnesemia
   D. Organophosphate poisoning
   E. Tick paralysis
   F. Snake envenomation (cobra, sea snake, coral snake, krait, mamba, viper, South American rattlesnake)
  V. Muscle
   A. Polymyositis/dermatomyositis
   B. Acid maltase deficiency (type II, Pompe's disease)
   C. Carnitine palmityl transferase deficiency
   D. Nemaline rod myopathy
   E. Hypokalemic periodic paralysis
   F. Hypophosphatemia
   G. Stonefish myotoxin
   H. Barium poisoning

SYMPTOMS ASSOCIATED WITH MINOR HEAD TRAUMA

I. Headache
II. Dizziness
III. Fatigue
IV. Reduced concentration
V. Memory deficit
VI. Irritability
VII. Anxiety
VIII. Insomnia
IX. Hyperacusis
X. Photophobia
XI. Depression
XII. Slowed information processing

(From Fisher JM: Cognitive and behavioral consequences of closed head injury. Semin Neurol 5:197–205, 1985, with permission.)

SYMPTOMS ASSOCIATED WITH MODERATE TO SEVERE HEAD TRAUMA

I. Behavioral problems
   A. Irritability
   B. Impulsivity
   C. Egocentricity
   D. Emotional lability
   E. Impaired judgment
   F. Impatience
   G. Tension or anxiety
   H. Depression
   I. Hypersexuality
   J. Hyposexuality
   K. Dependency
   L. Silliness or euphoria
   M. Aggressivity
   N. Apathy
   O. Childishness
   P. Disinhibition
II. Cognitive impairments
   A. Memory deficits
   B. Decreased abstraction
   C. Slowed information processing
   D. Poor concentration
   E. Deficits in processing and sequencing information
   F. Slowed reaction time
   G. Dysarthria
   H. Anomia
   I. Impaired auditory comprehension
   J. Decreased verbal fluency
   K. General intellectual deficits
   L. Planning or organizational problems

(From Fisher JM: Cognitive and behavioral consequences of closed head injury. Semin Neurol 5:197–204, 1985, with permission.)

THE CRITERIA FOR DETERMINATION
OF BRAIN DEATH

An individual with irreversible cessation of all functions of the entire brain, including the brainstem, is dead.

I. Cessation is recognized when evaluation discloses the following findings:
   A. Cerebral functions are absent
      1. Deep coma, cerebral unreceptivity, and unresponsivity
      2. Under some circumstances, confirmatory studies such as EEG or blood flow studies may be required
   B. Brainstem functions are absent
      1. Depends on reliable testing by experienced physician using adequate stimuli
      2. Pupillary light, corneal, oculocephalic (doll's eyes), oculovestibular (caloric testing), oropharyngeal, and respiratory (apnea) reflexes should be tested; if this is not possible, confirmatory tests are recommended

II. Irreversibility is recognized when evaluation discloses the following findings:
   A. The cause of the coma is established and is sufficient to account for the loss of brain function
   B. The possibility of recovery of any brain function is excluded (the most important reversible processes to recognize are sedation, hypothermia, neuromuscular blockade, and shock)
   C. The cessation of all brain function persists for an appropriate period of observation and/or trial of therapy
      1. In the absence of confirmatory tests, a period of at least 12 hours is recommended; in anoxic brain damage, the extent of the injury may be more difficult to assess and a period of 24 hours is recommended

(From Guidelines for the determination of death: report of the medical consultants on the diagnosis of death to the President's commission for the study of ethical problems in medicine and biomedical and behavioral research. Neurology 32:395–402, 1982, with permission.)

6

NEUROLOGICAL
DISEASES

Infectious Diseases of the
Nervous System

CNS INFECTION—DIFFERENTIAL DIAGNOSIS
BY ORGANISM

I. Bacterial
  - A. Meningococcus
  - B. *Haemophilus influenzae*
  - C. Pneumococcus
  - D. *Listeria*
  - E. *Staphylococcus*
  - F. *Streptococcus* group A
  - G. *Escherichia coli*, group B streptococcus in infants
  - H. Rickettsia
  - I. Tuberculosis
II. Viral
  - A. RNA
    1. Enterovirus
       a. Poliovirus
       b. Echovirus
  - C. Coxsackievirus
    2. Arbovirus (encephalitis)
       a. Eastern equine encephalitis
       b. Western equine encephalitis
       c. Venezuelan equine encephalitis
       d. St. Louis encephalitis
       e. Japanese encephalitis
       f. California encephalitis
       g. Tickborne encephalitis
       h. Colorado tick fever
    3. Influenza
    4. Measles
    5. Mumps
    6. Lymphocytic choriomeningitis
    7. Rabies
  - B. DNA
    1. Herpesvirus
       a. Simplex type I
       b. Varicella zoster
    2. CMV
    3. Epstein-Barr virus
    4. Adenovirus
  - C. "Slow virus"
    1. Progressive multifocal leukoencephalopathy
    2. Creutzfeldt-Jakob disease

List Continues

CNS INFECTION—DIFFERENTIAL DIAGNOSIS
BY ORGANISM (*Continued*)

      3. Subacute sclerosing panencephalitis
      4. Progressive rubella panencephalitis
      5. Kuru
   D. HIV
III. Fungal
   A. *Cryptococcus*
   B. Mucormycosis
   C. *Aspergillus*
   D. *Nocardia*
   E. Blastomycosis
   F. *Candida*
IV. Spirochetes
   A. Syphilis
   B. Lyme disease
 V. Parasitic
   A. Helminths (worms)
      1. Cysticercosis
      2. Trichinosis
      3. Schistosomiasis
      4. *Echinococcus* (hydatid cyst)
   B. Protozoa (unicellular)
      1. Toxoplasmosis
      2. Trypanosomiasis
      3. Malaria
      4. Amebiasis

INCIDENCE OF SELECTED PATHOGENS, BY AGE GROUP, IN BACTERIAL MENINGITIS

Pathogen	Incidence (percent)
Neonates	
Group B streptococcus	60
Escherichia coli and other gram-negative enteric organisms	30
Candida albicans	5
Listeria monocytogenes	2
Other	3
Staphylococcus aureus (and group B *Streptococcus*)—usually from skin, respiratory, or umbilical infections	
Pseudomonas or *Proteus*—usually from nursery	
Infants	
Haemophilus influenzae, type b	60
Neisseria meningiditis	25
Streptococcus pneumoniae	15
Adults	
Streptococcus pneumoniae	40
Neisseria meningiditis	30
Escherichia coli and other gram-negative enteric organisms	10
Listeria monocytogenes	5
Other	15

(Modified from Wood M, Anderson M: Neurological Infections. WB Saunders, Philadelphia, 1988, and Tureen JH, Sande MA: Acute bacterial infections of the central nervous system. pp. 559–575. In Aminoff MJ (ed.): Neurology and General Medicine, Churchill Livingstone, New York, 1989, with permission.)

BACTERIAL MENINGITIS: CAUSES BY ASSOCIATED FINDINGS

I. Petechial or purpuric rash
   A. Meningococcus
II. URI, otitis, sinusitis
   A. Pneumococcus
   B. *Haemophilus influenzae* anaerobes
III. Pneumonia
   A. Pneumococcus
   B. Meningococcus
IV. Critical care patient
   A. Gram-negative bacilli
   B. *Staphylococcus aureus*
V. Open skull fracture
   A. Gram-negative bacilli
   B. Staphylococci
VI. CSF rhinorrhea
   A. Pneumococcus
   B. Gram-negative bacilli
VII. Intracranial shunt
   A. *Staphylococcus epidermis*
VIII. Dermal sinus
   A. Gram-negative bacilli
   B. Staphylococci
IX. Endocarditis
   A. Pneumococcus
   B. *Staphylococcus aureus*

BACTERIAL MENINGITIS: CAUSES BY
ASSOCIATED FINDINGS (*Continued*)

   X. Immunosuppressed
     A. Gram-negative bacilli
     B. Fungi
  XI. Hyposplenism
     A. Pneumococcus
     B. *Haemophilus influenzae*
 XII. Alcoholism
     A. Pneumococcus
     B. *Listeria monocytogenes*
XIII. Diabetes mellitus
     A. Pneumococcus
     B. Gram-negative bacilli
     C. Staphylococci
 XIV. Leukemia
     A. Gram-negative bacilli
     B. *Staphylococcus aureus*
  XV. Lymphoma
     A. *Listeria monocytogenes*

(From Wood M, Anderson M: Acute purulent meningitis. pp. 44–133. In Neurological Infections. WB Saunders, Philadelphia, 1988, with permission.)

CONDITIONS ASSOCIATED WITH RECURRENT MENINGITIS

I. Bacterial infections
  A. Gross anatomical defects
    1. Traumatic
      a. Skull fracture involving the paranasal sinuses, cribriform plate, or petrous bone; postoperative, especially after nasal surgery
    2. Congential
      a. Myelomeningocele; midline cranial or spinal dermal sinus, with or without dermoid tumor; petrous fistula; neurenteric cysts
  B. Parameningeal focus of infection
    1. Otic with chronic mastoid osteomyelitis
    2. Paranasal sinusitis
    3. Brain abscess
    4. Cranial epidural abscess
    5. Spinal epidural abscess
    6. Subdural empyema
  C. Idiopathic recurrent bacterial meningitis
  D. Defective immune mechanisms
    1. Hypoimmunoglobulinemia
    2. Susceptibility in children after splenectomy
    3. Sickle cell anemia
    4. Chronic lymphocytic leukemia; multiple myeloma; lymphocytic lymphosarcoma
  E. Miscellaneous infections
    1. Brucellosis
    2. Leptospirosis
    3. Tuberculosis

CONDITIONS ASSOCIATED WITH RECURRENT
MENINGITIS (*Continued*)

II. Fungal infections
 A. Cryptococcosis
 B. Other fungal infections in case of treatment failure include blasto-
 mycosis, coccidioidomycosis, and histoplasmosis
III. Other infections
 A. Cerebral hydatid cyst
 B. Viruses
IV. Intracranial and intraspinal tumors
 A. Cerebral hemangioma (base of third ventricle)
 B. Ependymoma
 C. Epidermoid cyst
 D. Craniopharyngioma
 V. Etiology not established
 A. Sarcoidosis
 B. Behçet syndrome
 C. Vogt-Koyanagi-Harada syndrome
 D. Mollaret's meningitis

(From Hermans PE, Goldstein NP, Wellman WE: Mollaret's meningitis and
differential diagnosis of recurrent meningitis. Am J Med 52:128–139, 1972, with
permission.)

CSF PLEOCYTOSIS—PREDOMINANTLY POLYMORPHONUCLEAR CELLS

I. Infectious
  A. Bacterial meningitis (including syphilitic)
  B. Viral meningitis (early)
  D. Granulomatous meningoencephalitis
    1. Tuberculosis
    2. Histoplasmosis
  D. Parameningeal and parenchymal
    1. Cerebritis, brain abscess
    2. Subdural empyema
    3. Spinal epidural abscess
    4. Sphenoid sinusitis/abscess
  E. Septic emboli (infective endocarditis)

(From Leonard JM: Cerebrospinal fluid in patients with central nervous system infection. Neurol Clin 4:3–12, 1986, with permission.)

EMPIRIC THERAPY FOR PURULENT MENINGITIS

Age	Common Microorgansims	Therapy
0–4 wk	*Escherichia coli* Group B streptococci *Listeria monocytogenes*	Ampicillin plus a third-generation cephalosporin, or ampicillin plus an aminoglycoside
4–12 wk	*Escherichia coli* Group B streptococci *Listeria monocytogenes* *Haemophilus influenzae* *Streptococcus pneumoniae*	Ampicillin plus a third-generation cephalosporin
3 mo to 18 yr	*Haemophilus influenzae* *Neisseria meningitidis* *Streptococcus pneumoniae*	Third-generation cephalosporin, or ampicillin plus chloramphenicol
18–50 yr	*Streptococcus pneumoniae* *Neisseria meningitidis*	Penicillin G or ampicillin
Older than 50 yr	*Streptococcus pneumoniae* *Neisseria meningitidis* *Listeria monocytogenes* Gram-negative bacilli	Ampicillin plus a third-generation cephalosporin

(From Tunkel AR, Wispelwey B, Scheld WM: Bacterial meningitis: recent advances in pathophysiology and treatment. Ann Intern Med 112:610–621, 1989, with permission.)

ANTIMICROBIAL THERAPY FOR BACTERIAL MENINGITIS

Organism	Standard Therapy	Alternative Therapies
Neisseria meningitidis	Penicillin G or ampicillin	Third-generation cephalosporin, cefuroxime, chloramphenicol
Streptococcus pneumoniae	Penicillin G or ampicillin	Third-generation cephalosporin, cefuroxime, chloramphenicol
Haemophilus influenzae (beta-lactamase negative)	Ampicillin	Third-generation cephalosporin, cefuroxime, chloramphenicol
Haemophilus influenzae (beta-lactamase positive)	Third-generation cephalosporin	Cefuroxime, chloramphenicol
Enterobacteriaceae	Third-generation cephalosporin	Extended spectrum penicillin plus an aminoglycoside, aztreonam, quinolones
Pseudomonas aeruginosa	Ceftazidime (plus an aminoglycoside)	Extended spectrum penicillin plus an aminoglycoside, aztreonam, imipenem, quinolones
Streptococcus agalactiae	Penicillin G or ampicillin (plus an aminoglycoside)	Third-generation cephalosporin, chloramphenicol
Listeria monocytogenes	Ampicillin or penicillin G (plus an aminoglycoside)	Trimethoprim-sulfamethoxazole
Staphylococcus aureus (methicillin-sensitive)	Nafcillin or oxacillin	Vancomycin
Staphyloccus aureus (methicillin-resistant)	Vancomycin	Trimethoprim-sulfamethoxazole, quinolones
Staphylococcus epidermidis	Vancomycin (plus rifampin)	Teicoplanin, daptomycin

(From Tunkel AK, Wispelwey B, Scheld WM: Bacterial meningitis: recent advances in pathophysiology and treatment. Ann Intern Med 112:610–621, 1989, with permission.)

RECOMMENDED DOSES OF ANTIBIOTICS FOR BACTERIAL MENINGITIS IN ADULTS WITH NORMAL RENAL FUNCTION

Antibiotic	Daily Dose (per 24 h)	Dosing Interval (hr)
Penicillin G	20–24 million U	4
Ampicillin	12 g	4
Nafcillin, oxacillin	9–12 g	4
Chloramphenicol	4–6 g	6
Cefotaxime	12 g	4
Ceftizoxime	6–9 g	8
Ceftriaxone	4–6 g	12
Ceftazidime	6–12 g	8
Vancomycin	2 g	12
Gentamicin, tobramycin	3–4 mg/kg body weight	8
Amikacin	15 mg/kg body weight	8

(From Tunkel AR, Wispelwey B, Scheld WM: Bacterial meningitis: recent advances in pathophysiology and treatment. Ann Intern Med 112:610–621, 1989, with permission.)

IMPORTANT CAUSES OF ACUTE ENCEPHALITIS/ ENCEPHALOMYELITIS IN THE UNITED STATES

    I. Adenovirus
   II. Arenavirus
     A. Lymphocytic choriomeningitis*
  III. Bunyavirus
     A. California group* (LaCrosse virus)
  IV. Herpesvirus
     A. Simplex types 1 and 2
     B. Varicella zoster
     C. Epstein-Barr virus*
     D. CMV
   V. Orthomyxovirus
     A. Influenza types A* and B
  VI. Paramyxovirus
     A. Mumps*
     B. Measles
 VII. Picornavirus
     A. Poliovirus
     B. Coxsackie virus* types A and B
     C. Echovirus
VIII. Reovirus
     A. Colorado tick fever
  IX. Rhabdovirus
     A. Rabies*
   X. Togavirus
     A. Eastern equine encephalitis virus
     B. Western equine encephalitis virus
     C. Venezuelan equine encephalitis virus
     D. St. Louis encephalitis virus*
     E. Dengue
     F. Rubella

* Agents responsible for encephalitis in patients undergoing biopsy for presumed herpes simplex encephalitis.
(From Fishman MA: Pediatric Neurology. Grune & Stratton, Orlando, FL, 1986, with permission.)

SEASONAL PREVALENCE OF SOME VIRAL AGENTS

I. Summer and early fall
   A. St. Louis encephalitis
   B. California encephalitis
   C. Western equine encephalitis
   D. Eastern equine encephalitis
   E. Enteroviruses
   F. Rocky Mountain spotted fever (not viral)
II. Fall and winter
   A. Lymphocytic choriomeningitis virus
III. Winter and spring
   A. Mumps
IV. Year round
   A. Herpesvirus
   B. Epstein-Barr virus
   C. CMV
   D. *Leptospira* (not viral)
   E. Mycoplasma (not viral)

(From Tyler KL: Diagnosis and management of acute viral encephalitis. Semin Neurol 4:480–489, 1984, with permission.)

VIRUSES WITH LIMITED GEOGRAPHIC DISTRIBUTION IN THE UNITED STATES

I. Eastern equine encephalitis virus
   A. Atlantic and Gulf coasts
II. Venezuelan equine encephalitis virus
   A. Florida, Southwest
III. Colorado tick fever virus
   A. Rocky mountain states
IV. Powassan virus
   A. Northern United States and Canada
V. Rocky Mountain spotted fever (not viral)
   A. Mid and South Atlantic states

(From Tyler KL: Diagnosis and management of acute viral encephalitis. Semin Neurol 4:480–489, 1984, with permission.)

CLUES TO DIAGNOSIS OF SPECIFIC VIRAL AGENTS—LABORATORY EVALUATION

I. Leukopenia
   A. Lymphocytic choriomeningitis
   B. Colorado tick fever
   C. Epstein-Barr virus
   D. Venezuelan equine encephalitis
II. Thrombocytopenia
   A. Lymphocytic choriomeningitis
   B. Rocky Mountain spotted fever (not viral)
   C. Colorado tick fever
   D. St. Louis encephalitis (rare)
III. Anemia
   A. Mycoplasma
   B. Leptospirosis (occasional)
   C. Rocky Mountain spotted fever (occasional)
IV. Atypical lymphocytosis
   A. Epstein-Barr virus
   B. CMV
V. Renal dysfunction
   A. Leptospirosis
   B. St. Louis encephalitis
VI. Abnormal liver function
   A. Lymphocytic choriomeningitis
   B. Epstein-Barr virus
   C. Arboviruses (some)
   D. Mumps
   E. Leptospirosis
   F. Reye syndrome
VII. Increased creatine kinase, aldolase
   A. St. Louis encephalitis
   B. Rocky Mountain spotted fever (occasional)
VIII. Increased amylase, lipase
   A. Mumps, enterovirus (rare)
   B. Lymphocytic choriomeningitis (rare)
IX. Hyponatremia
   A. St. Louis encephalitis
   B. Rocky Mountain spotted fever

(From Tyler KL: Diagnosis and management of acute viral encephalitis. Semin Neurol 4:480–489, 1984, with permission.)

CLUES TO DIAGNOSIS OF SPECIFIC VIRAL AGENTS—CSF STUDIES

I. Decreased glucose (exclude tuberculosis, fungi, sarcoid, and neoplastic meningitis)
   A. Mumps
   B. Lymphocytic choriomeningitis
   C. Herpes simplex (late, rare)
   D. Leptospirosis (occasional)
II. Marked pleocytosis (>1,000 cells)
   A. Lymphocytic choriomeningitis
   B. Eastern equine encephalitis
   C. California encephalitis
   D. Mumps
III. PMNs predominate (after first 48 hours) (exclude bacterial meningitis, amebic meningitis, other nonviral causes)
   A. ECHO virus (especially E9)
   B. Eastern equine encephalitis
   C. Leptospirosis
   D. Acute hemorrhagic leukoencephalitis
IV. Red blood cells (nontraumatic tap) (exclude ameba, bacteria, nonviral causes)
   A. Herpes simplex
   B. California encephalitis
   C. Colorado tick fever virus
V. Atypical lymphocytes
   A. Epstein-Barr virus
   B. CMV

(From Tyler KL: Diagnosis and management of acute viral encephalitis. Semin Neurol 4:480–489, 1984, with permission.)

DISEASES THAT MIMIC VIRAL ENCEPHALITIS

I. Bacterial
   A. Leptospirosis
   B. Mycoplasma
   C. Tuberculosis
   D. Syphilis
   E. Brucellosis
   F. Typhoid fever
   G. Borreliosis
   H. Listeriosis
II. Fungal
   A. Cryptococcus
   B. Coccidiodomycosis
   C. Histoplasmosis
   D. Candidiasis
   E. Blastomycosis
III. Parasitic
   A. Toxoplasmosis
   B. Cysticercosis
   C. Trichinosis
   D. Echinococcosis
   E. Trypanosomiasis
   F. Malaria
   G. Amebiasis

DISEASES THAT MIMIC VIRAL ENCEPHALITIS
(*Continued*)

IV. Chlamydial and rickettsial
  A. Rocky mountain spotted fever
  B. Typhus
  C. Lymphogranuloma venereum
 V. Post- or parainfectious
  A. Acute disseminated encephalomyelitis
  B. Reye syndrome
VI. Neoplasia
  A. Carcinomatous meningitis
  B. Lymphoma
  C. Leukemia
VII. Miscellaneous
  A. Acute "toxic" and "metabolic" encephalopathy
  B. Acute hemorrhagic encephalitis
  C. Sarcoidosis
  D. Behçet's disease
  E. CNS vasculitis
  F. Parameningeal infection (mastoiditis, osteomyelitis)
  G. Whipple's disease

(Modified from Tyler KL: Diagnosis and management of acute viral encephalitis. Semin Neurol 4:480–489, 1984, with permission.)

CLINICAL MANIFESTATIONS OF LYME DISEASE

I. Meningoencephalitis syndrome (acute or chronic)
   A. Headache
   B. Stiff neck
   C. Lethargy
   D. Irritability
   E. Change in mental status/dementia
   F. Seizures
II. Peripheral neuropathy
   A. Mononeuritis
   B. Mononeuritis multiplex
   C. Radiculopathy
   D. Lumbar or brachial plexitis
   E. Distal axonal neuropathy
   F. Demyelinating neuropathy
   G. Carpal tunnel syndrome
III. Focal myositis
IV. Cranial neuropathy
   A. CN VII most common
   B. May also see CN IV, V, VI, and VIII
V. Multiple sclerosis-like disease
VI. Transverse myelitis
VII. Psychiatric disease
VIII. Chronic fatigue syndrome
IX. Less common:
   A. Pseudotumor cerebri
   B. Chorea

CHRONIC MENINGITIS

I. Infectious
  A. Common
    1. *Mycobacterium tuberculosis*
    2. *Cryptococcus neoformans*
    3. *Histoplasma capsulatum*
    4. *Candida* sp
    5. *Aspergillus* sp
    6. *Blastomyces dermatitidis*
    7. *Treponema pallidum*
    8. *Brucella* sp
    9. *Toxoplasma gondii*
    10. *Nocardia asteroides*
    11. *Actinomyces* sp
    12. Dermatomyces
    13. *Taenia solium*
    14. *Borrelia burgdorferi* (Lyme disease)
    15. *Streptococcus* sp (infective endocarditis)
  B. Rare
    1. *Pseudoallescheria boydii*
    2. *Sporothrix schenckii*
    3. *Zygomycetes* sp
    4. *Coenurus cerebralis*
    5. *Leptospira icterohaemorrhagiae*
    6. *Angiostrongylus cantonensis* and other worms
    7. Coccidiomycoses
II. Noninfectious causes
  A. Neoplasm
    1. Metastatic carcinomatous meningitis
    2. Lymphomatous meningitis
    3. Leukemic meningitis
    4. Meningeal gliomatosis
  B. Vasculitis
  C. Vogt-Koyanagi-Harada syndrome
  D. Chronic benign lymphocytic meningitis
  E. Sarcoidosis
  F. Systemic lupus erythematosus
  G. Behçet syndrome
  H. Mollaret's meningitis
  I. Whipple's disease

(From Wood M, Anderson M: Chronic meningitis. p. 169–248. In Neurological Infections. WB Saunders, Philadelphia, 1988, with permission.)

NEUROLOGICAL COMPLICATIONS OF AIDS

I. CNS
  A. Primary HIV infection
    1. Aseptic meningitis
    2. Subacute encephalopathy/AIDS dementia
    3. Vacuolar myelopathy
    4. Vasculitis
  B. Opportunistic infections
    1. Viral
      a. Cytomegalovirus (retinitis, encephalitis)
      b. Progressive multifocal leukoencephalopathy
      c. Herpes simplex virus types I and II
      d. Varicella zoster virus
    2. Nonviral
      a. *Toxoplasma gondii*
      b. *Cryptococcus neoformans*
      c. *Mycobacterium*
      d. *Aspergillus fumigatus*
      e. *Histoplasma capsulatum*
      f. *Nocardia asteroides*
      g. Mucormycosis
      h. Neurosyphilis
  C. Neoplasms
    1. Primary CNS lymphoma
    2. Metastatic systemic lymphoma
    3. Metastatic Kaposi sarcoma
    4. Lymphomatous meningitis
II. Neuromuscular syndromes
  A. Neuropathies
    1. Acute inflammatory demyelinating polyneuropathy
    2. Chronic inflammatory demyelinating polyneuropathy
    3. Mononeuritis multiplex
    4. Progressive polyradiculopathy
    5. Distal symmetric sensorimotor polyneuropathy
  B. Myopathies
    1. Polymyositis
    2. Nemaline rod myopathy
    3. Zidovudine-induced myopathy

(Modified from Kieburtz K, Schiffer RB: Neurologic manifestations of human immunodeficiency virus infections. Neurol Clin 7:447–468, 1989, with permission.)

Neuro-oncology

CLASSIFICATION OF BRAIN TUMORS

I. Tumors of neuroglial cells
    A. Astrocytoma
    B. Glioblastoma multiforme
    C. Oligodendroglioma
    D. Ependymoma, subependymoma
II. Tumors of neuronal cells and primitive precursors
    A. Medulloblastoma
    B. Ganglioglioma
    C. Neuroblastoma
III. Tumors of mesodermal origin
    A. Meningioma/meningiosarcoma
IV. Tumors of cranial nerves
    A. Schwannoma
V. Tumors of reticuloendothelial system
    A. Primary CNS lymphoma
    B. Histiocytoses
    C. Leukemias
VI. Tumors of the choriod plexus and related structures
    A. Choroid plexus papilloma/carcinoma
VII. Tumors of the pineal region
    A. Germinoma
    B. Teratoma
    C. Embryonal cell carcinoma/choriocarcinoma
    D. Pineoblastoma
    E. Glioma
VIII. Tumors of vascular origin
    A. Hemangioblastoma
    B. Cavernous angioma
IX. Developmental tumors/tumor-like lesions
    A. Craniopharyngioma
    B. Lipoma
    C. Dermoid/epidermoid cyst
    D. AVMs
X. Local tumors
    A. Pituitary adenoma
    B. Chordoma
    C. Chemodectoma
    D. Nasopharyngeal carcinoma
    E. Orbital tumors

List Continues

CLASSIFICATION OF BRAIN TUMORS *(Continued)*

XI. Metastatic tumors
- A. Lung
- B. Breast
- C. Melanoma
- D. Kidney
- E. GI (especially colorectal)
- F. Prostate
- G. Thyroid

(From Polachini I: Brain tumors: MR imaging. pp. 39–50. In: American Academy of Neurology, Annual Course #242 (Clinical Neuroimaging), 1990, with permission.)

TOPOGRAPHIC DIFFERENTIAL DIAGNOSIS OF INTRACRANIAL TUMORS IN ADULTHOOD—SUPRATENTORIAL

I. Cerebral hemisphere
   A. Astrocytoma
   B. Glioblastoma multiforme
   C. Meningioma
   D. Metastatic
   E. Cavernous angioma
   F. Oligodendroglioma
   G. Ganglioglioma
   H. Primary CNS lymphoma
   I. Ependymoma
   J. Sarcoma

II. Corpus callosum
   A. Glioblastoma multiforme
   B. Astrocytoma
   C. Oligodendrioglioma
   D. Metastatic
   E. Lipoma

III. Lateral ventricle
   A. Ependymoma
   B. Meningioma
   C. Subependymoma
   D. Choroid plexus papilloma/carcinoma

IV. Region of the third ventricle
   A. Pilocytic astrocytoma/astrocytoma
   B. Colloid cyst
   C. Ependymoma
   D. Oligodendroglioma

V. Optic chiasm and nerve
   A. Meningioma
   B. Astrocytoma

VI. Pituitary region
   A. Adenoma
   B. Craniopharyngioma
   C. Meningioma
   D. Germ cell neoplasm
   E. Dermoid cyst

List Continues

TOPOGRAPHIC DIFFERENTIAL DIAGNOSIS OF INTRACRANIAL TUMORS IN ADULTHOOD— SUPRATENTORIAL *(Continued)*

VII. Pineal region
    A. Germ cell neoplasm
    B. Teratoma
    C. Pineocytoma/pineoblastoma
    D. Epidermoid cyst

(From Polachini I: Brain tumors: MR imaging. pp. 39–50. In: American Academy of Neurology, Annual Course #242 (Clinical Neuroimaging), 1990, with permission.)

TOPOGRAPHIC DIFFERENTIAL DIAGNOSIS OF INTRACRANIAL TUMORS IN ADULTHOOD— INFRATENTORIAL

I. Cerebellum
   A. Hemangioblastoma
   B. Metastatic
   C. Astrocytoma
   D. Cavernous angioma
   E. Medulloblastoma
II. Cerebellopontine angle
   A. Acoustic schwannoma
   B. Meningioma
   C. Epidermoid cyst
   D. Nonacoustic (CN V, VII, IX, X, XI, XII) schwannoma
   E. Paraganglioma
   F. Choroid plexus papilloma
   G. Ependymoma
   H. Metastatic tumor
III. Fourth ventricle
   A. Ependymoma
   B. Choroid plexus papilloma
   C. Subependymoma
   D. Meningioma
IV. Region of the foramen magnum
   A. Meningioma
   B. Schwannoma
   C. Neurofibroma
V. Brainstem
   A. Metastatic
   B. Venous angioma
   C. Astrocytoma-anaplastic astrocytoma

(From Polachini I: Brain tumors: MR imaging. pp. 39–50. In: American Academy of Neurology, Annual Course #242 (Clinical Neuroimaging), 1990, with permission.)

BRAIN METASTASIS

I. Brain metastasis by primary site (e.g., of every 100 patients with brain metastases, the most common source will be lung)
    A. Lung
    B. Breast
    C. Melanoma
    D. Gastrointestinal tract (liver, colon, and rectum)
    E. Kidney
    F. Leukemia
    G. Reproductive (testicular, uterus, ovarian)
    H. Sarcoma
    I. Endocrine (thyroid)

II. Neoplasms prone to go to the brain (e.g., of every 100 patients with melanoma, 75 will develop metastases to the brain)
    A. Melanomas (75%)
    B. Testicular tumors (60%)
    C. Bronchiogenic carcinoma (35%)
    D. Lymphoma (20%)
    E. Renal (15%)

III. Tumors that often spread within the CNS
    A. Glioblastoma
    B. Oligodendroglioma
    C. Lymphoma
    D. Medulloblastoma
    E. Ependymoblastoma

PARANEOPLASTIC SYNDROMES

I. Brain
    A. Limbic encephalitis
    B. Photoreceptor degeneration
    C. Progressive multifocal leukoencephalopathy
    D. Optic neuritis
II. Cerebellum/brainstem
    A. Paraneoplastic subacute cerebellar degeneration
    B. Bulbar encephalitis
    C. Opsoclonus/myoclonus
III. Spinal cord
    A. Necrotizing myelopathy
    B. Subacute motor neuronopathy
IV. Peripheral nerve
    A. Subacute sensorimotor neuropathy
    B. Subacute sensory neuronopathy
    C. Subacute motor neuropathy
    D. Paraproteinemic neuropathy (e.g., myeloma, Waldenström's macroglobulinemia, benign monoclonal gammopathy)
    E. Motor neuropathy with insulinoma
    F. Guillain-Barré syndrome
V. Neuromuscular junction
    A. Myasthenia gravis
    B. Eaton-Lambert syndrome
VI. Muscle
    A. Polymyositis/dermatomyositis
    B. Carcinoid myopathy
    C. Muscle weakness

PSEUDOTUMOR CEREBRI

The following is a list of diseases known to produce papilledema and increased intracranial pressure (excluding space-occupying intracranial lesions).

 I. Renal diseases
  A. Chronic uremia
 II. Developmental diseases
  A. Syringomyelia
  B. Craniostenosis
  C. Aqueductal stenosis (adult type)
 III. Toxic conditions
  A. Heavy metal poisoning (lead, arsenic)
  B. Hypervitaminosis A
  C. Tetracycline therapy
  D. Nalidixic acid therapy
  E. Prolonged steroid therapy
  F. Steroid withdrawal
 IV. Allergic diseases
  A. Serum sickness
  B. Allergies
 V. Infectious diseases
  A. Bacterial (subacute bacterial endocarditis)
  B. Meningitis
  C. Chronic mastoiditis (lateral-sinus thrombosis)
  D. Brucellosis
 VI. Viral diseases
  A. Poliomyelitis
  B. Acute lymphocytic meningitis
  C. Coxsackie B virus encephalitis
  D. Inclusion body encephalitis
  E. Recurrent polyneuritis
  F. Guillain-Barré syndrome
 VII. Parasitic diseases
  A. Sandfly fever
  B. Trypanosomiasis
  C. Torulosis
 VIII. Metabolic endocrine conditions
  A. Eclampsia
  B. Hypoparathyroidism
  C. Addison's disease
  D. Scurvy
  E. Oral progestational agents

PSEUDOTUMOR CEREBRI (*Continued*)

    F. Diabetic ketoacidosis
    G. Menarche
    H. Obesity
    I. Menstrual abnormalities
    J. Pregnancy
  IX. Degenerative diseases
    A. Schilder's disease
    B. Muscular dystrophy
   X. Miscellaneous diseases
    A. Gastrointestinal hemorrhage
    B. Lupus erythematosus
    C. Sarcoidosis
    D. Syphilis
    E. Subarachnoid hemorrhage
    F. Status epilepticus
    G. Paget's disease
    H. Opticochiasmatic arachnoiditis
  XI. Neoplastic diseases
    A. Leukemia
    B. Spinal cord tumors
 XII. Hematological diseases
    A. Infectious mononucleosis
    B. Idiopathic thrombocytopenic purpura
    C. Pernicious anemia
    D. Polycythemia
    E. Iron-deficient anemia
    F. Hemophilia
XIII. Circulatory diseases
    A. Congestive heart failure
    B. Mediastinal neoplasm
    C. Congenital cardiac lesion
    D. Hypertensive encephalopathy
    E. Pulmonary emphysema
    F. Dural-sinus thrombosis
    G. Chronic pulmonary hypoventilaton

(From Rothner DA, Brust JM: Pseudotumor cerebri. Arch Neurol 30:110–112, 1974, with permission.)

Cerebrovascular Disease

COMMON SYMPTOMS AND SIGNS OF STROKE

    I. Pure motor paresis
   II. Pure sensory abnormalities
  III. Sensory and motor abnormalities
  IV. Motor disturbances other than partial paralysis or hemiplegia (ataxis, incoordination, tremor, dystonia)
    V. Language or speech disturbance (if not due to coma or overt dementia)
  VI. Other higher cortical dysfunction (anmesia, agnosia, apraxia, confusion, delerium, dementia)
 VII. Visual symptoms (loss of vision, blurring of vision, diplopia)
VIII. Vertigo, dizziness, unsteadiness
  IX. Swallowing impairment
    X. Hearing loss, tinnitus
  XI. Convulsions, epileptic seizures
 XII. Loss of consciousness
XIII. Loss of sphincter control (if not due to seizures or coma)
XIV. Headache
 XV. Nausea and vomiting
XVI. Neck stiffness
XVII. Additional signs found at examination include brisk jerk reflexes, Babinski sign, decerebrate or decorticate signs, nystagmus

(From Report of the WHO Task Force on Stroke and Other Cerebrovascular Disorders: Stroke—1989: recommendations on stroke prevention, diagnosis, and therapy. Stroke 20:1407–1431, 1989, with permission.)

STROKE RISK FACTORS AND PREVENTION

I. Characteristics and lifestyle
  A. Definite
    1. Cigarette smoking
    2. Alcohol consumption
    3. Drug abuse
    4. Age (increasing)
    5. Sex (male > female)
    6. Race (blacks > whites)
    7. Familial factors
  B. Possible
    1. Oral contraceptive use
    2. Diet (e.g., cholesterol, fats)
    3. Personality type (e.g., type A)
    4. Geographical location (e.g., Southeastern U.S.)
    5. Season (e.g., low in summer, peak in early winter)
    6. Climate (? colder ambient temperature)
    7. Socioeconomic factors (greater risk in lower socioeconomic class)
    8. Physical inactivity
    9. Obesity
    10. Abnormal blood lipids
    11. Maternal death due to stroke
II. Disease or disease markers
  A. Definite
    1. Hypertension
    2. Cardiac disease
    3. TIA
    4. Elevated hematocrit
    5. Diabetes mellitus
    6. Sickle cell disease
    7. Elevated fibrinogen concentration
    8. Migraine and migraine equivalents
  B. Possible
    1. Hyperuricemia
    2. Hypothyroidism
III. Asymptomatic lesions
  A. Physical examination
    1. Bruit (cervical, orbital, cranial)
    2. Retinal emboli
    3. Blood pressure differences between arms
    4. Reduced pressure on oculoplethysmography

STROKE RISK FACTORS AND PREVENTION
(*Continued*)

B. Imaging
   1. Silent infarction or hemorrhage (MRI or CT)
   2. AVM, aneurysm, hematoma
   3. Atherosclerosis with arterial stenosis
   4. Fibromuscular dysplasia, dissection
IV. Multiple factors in combination

(From Report of the National Institute of Neurological Disorders and Stroke: Classification of cerebrovascular diseases III. Stroke 21:637–676, 1990, with permission.)

SYMPTOMS NOT USUALLY CONSIDERED A TIA

    I. March of a sensory deficit
   II. Vertigo alone
  III. Dizziness (or wooziness) alone
  IV. Dysphagia alone
   V. Dysarthria alone
  VI. Diplopia alone
 VII. Incontinence of bowel or bladder
VIII. Loss of vision associated with alteration of level of consciousness
  IX. Focal symptoms associated with migraines
   X. Confusion alone
  XI. Amnesia alone
 XII. Drop attacks alone
XIII. Unconsciousness without other signs of posterior (vertebrobasilar) circulation symptoms
XIV. Tonic and/or clonic activity
 XV. Prolonged march of symptoms over several areas of the body
XVI. Scintillating scotoma

(From Report of the National Institute of Neurological Disorders and Stroke: Classification of cerebrovascular diseases III. Stroke 21:637–676, 1990, with permission.)

DISORDERS THAT CAN MIMIC A TIA

    I. Migraine
   II. Seizure (partial)
  III. Hypoglycemia
   IV. Subdural hematoma
    V. Intracerebral hematoma
   VI. Subarachnoid hemorrhage
  VII. Cerebral infarction
 VIII. Tumor
   IX. Arteriovenous malformation
    X. Demyelinating disease (multiple sclerosis)
   XI. Incipient syncope
  XII. Orthostatic hypotension
 XIII. Cardiac arrhythmia
  XIV. Amnestic syndrome
   XV. Narcolepsy
  XVI. Cataplexy
 XVII. Intracranial inflammation
XVIII. Periodic paralysis
  XIX. Pressure neuropathy
   XX. Dizziness of uncertain etiology
  XXI. Anxiety
 XXII. Hyperventilation
XXIII. Labyrynthine disease

(From Reggia JA, Tabb R, Price TR, et al: Computer-aided assessment of transient ischemic attacks: a clinical evaluation. Arch Neurol 41:1248–1254, 1984 with permission.)

CAUSES OF INFARCTION IN 100 YOUNG ADULTS

	No. of Cases	Total
Cerebrovascular atherosclerosis		**18**
Cerebral embolism		
Previously known cardiac disease (e.g., rheumatic heart disease, valve prosthesis)		**23**
Previously unrecognized source		**8**
Left atrial myxoma	2	
Pulmonary arteriovenous malformation	2	
Atrial septal defect	2	
Occult mitral stenosis	1	
Idiopathic cardiomyopathy	1	
Nonatherosclerotic cerebral vasculopathy (angiographic diagnosis)		**10**
Spontaneous carotid dissection	2	
Following neck irradiation	3	
Idiopathic venous sinus thrombosis	1	
Cerebral vasculitis	2	
Vertebral artery injury secondary to neck turning	2	
Coagulopathy and systemic inflammation (serological diagnosis)		**9**
SLE with/without lupus anticoagulant	4	
Lupus anticoagulant without SLE	1	
Homocystinuria	1	
Systemic vasculitis	1	
Coagulopathy with thrombocytopenia (unclassified)	1	
Severe Crohn's disease	1	
Peripartum		**5**
Uncertain etiology		**27**
Associated with migraine only	5	
Associated with oral contraceptive use only	2	
Migraine and oral contraceptive use	7	
Mitral valve prolapse only	3	
"Idiopathic"/no association	10	

(From Hart RG, Miller VT: Cerebral infarcts in young adults: a practical approach. Stroke 14:110–114, 1983, with permission.)

DIFFERENTIAL DIAGNOSIS OF CEREBRAL INFARCTION IN YOUNG ADULTS

I. Cerebrovascular atherosclerosis (thrombotic or embolic)
II. Embolism
    A. Cardiac source
        1. Valvular (mitral stenosis, prosthetic valve, infective endocarditis, marantic endocarditis, Libman-Sacks endocarditis, mitral annulus calcification, mitral valve prolapse, calcific aortic stenosis)
        2. Atrial fibrillation and sick sinus syndrome
        3. Acute myocardial infarction and/or left ventricular aneurysm
        4. Left atrial myxoma
        5. Cardiomyopathy
    B. Paradoxical embolism or pulmonary source
        1. Pulmonary arteriovenous malformation (including Osler-Weber-Rendu disease)
        2. Atrial and ventricular septal defects with R→L shunt
        3. Patent foramen ovale with shunt
        4. Pulmonary vein thrombosis
        5. Pulmonary and mediastinal tumors
    C. Other
        1. Aortic cholesterol embolism
        2. Transient embologenic aortitis
        3. Emboli distal to unruptured aneurysm
        4. Fat embolism syndrome
III. Arteriopathy
    A. Inflammatory (see also vasculitis classification)
        1. Takayasu's disease
        2. Allergic (Churg-Strauss syndrome) and granulomatous
        3. Infective—specific: syphilis, mucormycosis, ophthalmic zoster, TB, malaria; nonspecific: severe tonsillitis or lymphadenitis
        4. Associated with drug use (e.g., amphetamine, cocaine, phenylpropanolamine)
        5. Associated with systemic disease (lupus, Wegener's granulomatosis, polyarteritis nodosa, rheumatoid arthritis, Sjögren syndrome, scleroderma, Dego's disease, Behçet syndrome, acute rheumatic fever, inflammatory bowel disease)
    B. Noninflammatory
        1. Spontaneous dissection
        2. Post-therapeutic irradiation
        3. Fibromuscular hyperplasia
        4. Moyamoya disease and progressive arterial occlusion syndrome
        5. Congophilic (amyloid) angiopathy

DIFFERENTIAL DIAGNOSIS OF CEREBRAL INFARCTION IN YOUNG ADULTS (*Continued*)

    6. Thromboangiitis obliterans

    7. Familial: homocystinuria, Fabry's disease, pseudoxanthoma elasticum

IV. Vasospasm associated with the following:

  A. Migraine

  B. Subarachnoid hemorrhage

  C. Hypertensive encephalopathy

  D. Cerebral arteriography

 V. Hematological disease and coagulopathies

  A. Hyperviscosity

    1. Polycythemia and myeloproliferative dysproteinemia (myeloma, Waldenström's macroglobulinemia, cryoglobulinemia)

  B. Coagulopathy

    1. Thrombotic thrombocytopenia purpura

    2. Chronic diffuse intravasculara coagulation

    3. Paroxysmal nocturnal hemoglobinuria

    4. Oral contraceptive use/peripartum/pregnancy

    5. Thrombocythemia

    6. Sickle cell and hemoglobin C disease

    7. Lupus anticoagulant

    8. Nephrotic syndrome

    9. C_2 complement deficiency (familial)

    10. Protein C deficiency (familial)

  C. Controversial associations

    1. Platelet hyperaggregability

    2. Fibrinolytic insufficiency

    3. Increased factor VIII

    4. Antithrombin III deficiency

    5. Vitamin K and antifibrinolytic therapy

    6. Acute alcohol intoxication

VI. Miscellaneous

    1. Trauma (direct, indirect, rotation, and extension injuries)

    2. Mechanical (cervical rib, atlantoaxial subluxation)

    3. Related to systemic hypotension

    4. Iatrogenic (perioperative and periprocedural, including air and foreign particle embolism)

    5. Cortical sinus or vein thrombosis

(From Hart RG, Miller VT: Cerebral infarcts in young adults: a practical approach. Stroke 14:110–114, 1983, with permission.)

SIGNS AND SYMPTOMS OF ISCHEMIA IN THE ANTERIOR CIRCULATION

 I. Ophthalmic artery
    A. Monocular blindness
 II. Anterior cerebral artery
    A. Weakness contralateral side (leg > arm, face)
    B. Sensory loss of contralateral side (leg > arm, face)
    C. Eye deviation toward side of infarction
    D. Apraxia (left hand)
    E. Memory loss
    F. Incontinence
    G. Agraphia (left side)
    H. Bradykinesia
     I. Tactile anomia (left side)
    J. Behavioral changes (akinetic mutism, bilateral infarction, abulia, loss of interest and initiative)
    K. Reduction in spontaneous speech
    L. Hand/foot groping and grasping
III. Middle cerebral artery
    A. Contralateral hemiplegia (face, arm > leg)
    B. Contralateral sensory loss (face, arm > leg)
    C. Aphasia (left hemisphere)
    D. Hemianopia
    E. Deviation of eyes and head to side of infarction
    F. Neglect (right hemisphere > left)
    G. Apraxia (left hemisphere)
    H. Impaired optokinetic responses
     I. Contructional/spacial defects (right hemisphere)
    J. Hemi-inattention (right hemisphere > left)
    K. Impersistence
    L. Amusia (right hemisphere)
    M. Aprosody (right hemisphere)
    N. Prosopagnosia (right hemisphere)
    O. Delirium (distraction by irrelevant stimuli)
    P. Limb shaking (with TIA)

SIGNS AND SYMPTOMS OF ISCHEMIA IN THE POSTERIOR CIRCULATION

I. Symptoms
   A. Dizziness
   B. Gait ataxia
   C. Inability to stand
   D. Bilateral limb weakness
   E. Alternating weakness on both sides of the body
   F. Bilateral numbness
   G. Crossed weakness
   H. Diplopia
   I. Crossed paresthesias or numbness
   J. Bilateral loss of vision
   K. Poor memory
   L. Tinnitus or deafness
   M. Difficulty seeing to one side
   N. Occipital or neck ache

II. Signs
   A. Nystagmus
   B. Vertical gaze palsy
   C. Dysconjugate gaze
   D. Internuclear ophthalmoplegia
   E. Ocular skew
   F. Bilateral limb weakness
   G. Crossed motor weakness (ipsilateral CN VII, VI, XII palsy and contralateral hemiparesis)
   H. Crossed sensory loss (ipsilateral face and contralateral body)
   I. Unilateral gaze palsy with contralateral hemiparesis
   J. CN VI or III palsy
   K. Hemianopsia or bilateral hemianopsia
   L. Amnesia

(From Caplan LR: Transient ischemic attacks and stroke in the distribution of the vertebrobasilar system: clinical manifestations. pp. 103–129. In Moore WS: Surgery for Cerebrovascular Disease. Churchill Livingstone, New York, 1987, with permission.)

CLINICAL FEATURES OF LATERAL MEDULLARY INFARCT

I. Characteristic
   A. Dysphagia
   B. Dysarthria
   C. Horner syndrome
   D. Crossed sensory loss
   E. Ipsilateral facial weakness
II. Common
   A. Headaches
   B. Nausea and vomiting
   C. Ipsilateral facial pain
   D. Ipsilateral facial numbness
   E. Ipsilateral limb ataxia
   F. Gait ataxia
   G. Lateropulsion
   H. Diplopia (horizontal or vertical)
III. Occasional
   A. Hiccups
   B. Nystagmus
   C. Ipsilateral Babinski sign
   D. Carotid sinus hypersensitivity

(From Heros RC: Cerebral hemorrhage and infarction. Stroke 13:106–109, 1982, with permission.)

LACUNAR SYNDROMES

    I. Pure sensory stroke
   II. Pure motor hemiparesis (PMH)
  III. Ataxic hemiparesis
   IV. Dysarthria-clumsy hand syndrome
    V. Modified PMH with "motor aphasia"
   VI. PMH sparing face
  VII. Mesencephalothalamic syndrome (CN III, paresis of vertical gaze, and abulia)
 VIII. Thalamic dementia
   IX. PMH with horizontal gaze palsy
    X. PMH with crossed third-nerve palsy (Weber syndrome)
   XI. PMH with crossed sixth-nerve palsy
  XII. PMH with confusion
 XIII. Cerebellar ataxia with crossed third-nerve palsy (Claude syndrome)
  XIV. Sensorimotor stroke (thalamocapsular)
   XV. Hemiballismus
  XVI. Lower basilar branch syndrome (dizziness, diplopia, gaze palsy, dysarthria, cerebellar ataxia, trigeminal numbness)
 XVII. Lateral medullary syndrome (Wallenberg syndrome)
XVIII. Lateral pontomedullary syndrome
  XIX. Loss of memory(?)
   XX. Locked-in syndrome (bilateral PMH)
  XXI. Miscellaneous
       A. Weakness of one leg with ease of falling
       B. Pure dysarthria
       C. Acute dystonia of thalamic origin

Note: Syndromes I–IV are the most common. See separate list for details. (From Fisher CM: Lacunar stroke and infarcts: a review. Neurology 32:871–876, 1982, with permission.)

ANATOMICAL LOCATION OF COMMON LACUNAR SYNDROMES

Lacunar Syndrome	Usual Location of Infarct	Clinical Deficit
Pure motor hemiparesis	Contralateral internal capsule or basis pontis	Paresis of face, arm, and leg
Pure sensory stroke	Contralateral thalamus	Paresthesias of face, arm, and leg
Dysarthria-clumsy hand syndrome	Contralateral internal capsule or basis pontis	Dysarthria and hemiataxia
Ataxic hemiparesis	Contralateral internall capsule or basis pontis	Mild hemiparesis and ipsilateral ataxia

CAUSES OF CAROTID DISSECTION ASSOCIATED WITH MILD TRAUMA

   I. Coughing
  II. Brushing teeth
 III. Nose blowing
  IV. Chiropractic manipulation
   V. Head-turning during a parade
  VI. Sports activities (tennis, skiing, basketball, volleyball, polo, football, bowling, swimming, hockey)
 VII. Old whiplash injury
VIII. Car sliding on ice
  IX. Intraoral trauma (fall with object in mouth)
   X. Motor vehicle accident
  XI. Neck flexing with child abuse (scolding)
 XII. Chewing
XIII. Straightening up after bending
 XIV. Trampoline exercises
  XV. "Head banging" during dancing
 XVI. Strangulation
XVII. Childbirth
XVIII. "Downing" shots of liquor
 XIX. Intercourse

CAUSES OF CARDIOGENIC CEREBRAL EMBOLISM

I. Common sources
  A. Atrial fibrillation
  B. Acute myocardial infarction (AMI)
  C. Ventricular thrombi and aneurysm remote from AMI
  D. Nonischemic cardiomyopathy
  E. Mitral valve prolapse
  F. Prosthetic cardiac valves
  G. Nonbacterial thrombotic endocarditis
  H. Infective endocarditis
  I. Mitral annulus calcification
  J. Calcific aortic stenosis
II. Less common sources
  A. Nonischemic cardiomyopathies
    1. Hypertrophic
    2. Amyloid
    3. Rheumatic myocarditis
    4. Neuromuscular disorders
    5. Catecholamine induced
    6. Doxorubicin HCl (Adriamycin)
    7. Idiopathic
    8. Viral
    9. Peripartum
    10. Confusion
    11. Hypereosinophilic
    12. Alcoholic
    13. Chagas disease
  B. Ventricular thrombi without underlying cardiac disease
    1. Polycystic disease
    2. Myeloproliferative disorders/thrombocythemia
    3. System lupus
    4. Malignancy
    5. Idiopathic
  C. Inflammatory valvulitis: Libman-Sacks endocarditis, Behçet syndrome
  D. Atrial septal aneurysms
  E. Aortic aneurysms
  F. Paradoxical emboli
    1. Atrial septal defects
    2. Patent foramen ovale
    3. Ventricular septal defects
    4. Pulmonary arteriovenous fistulas
  G. Cardiac tumors: primary and metastatic

(Modified from Cerebral Embolism Task Force: Cardiogenic brain embolism: the second report of the Cerebral Embolism Task Force. Arch Neurol 46:727–743, 1989, with permission.)

CAUSES OF CEREBRAL VENOUS THROMBOSIS

I. Changes in the constituents of the blood
   A. Antithrombin III deficiency
   B. Oral contraceptives
   C. Ulcerative colitis
   D. Polycythemia
   E. Crohn's disease
   F. Hemolytic anemia
   G. Pregnancy and puerperium
   H. Leukemia
   I. Paroxysmal nocturnal hemoglobinuria
   J. Carcinoma
   K. Idiopathic thrombocytosis
   L. Nephrotic syndrome
   M. Androgen therapy
   N. Cryofibrinogenemia
   O. Disseminated intravascular coagulation
   P. Behçet syndrome
II. Changes in the wall
   A. Carcinoma (invasion)
   B. Lymphoma (invasion)
   C. Behçet syndrome
   D. Arteriovenous malformation
   E. Sarcoidosis
   F. Leukemia (invasion)
   G. Meningitis
   H. Chronic otitis media
   I. Wegener's granulomatosis
   J. Aspergillosis
   K. Mastoiditis

CAUSES OF CEREBRAL VENOUS THROMBOSIS
(*Continued*)

III. Changes in the blood flow and miscellaneous
   - A. Cardiac failure
   - B. Cachexia and marasmus
   - C. Post-traumatic changes
   - D. Cerebral artery thrombosis
   - E. Chronic obstructive airway disease
   - F. Trichinosis
   - G. Transvenous pacemaker
   - H. Dehydration/hyperpyrexia
   - I. Congenital heart disease
   - J. Budd-Chiari syndrome
   - K. Idiopathic changes

(From Gates PC, Barnett HJM: Venous disease: cortical veins and sinuses. pp. 707–719. In: Barnett HJM, Mohr JP, Stein BM, Yatsu FM: Stroke. Churchill Livingstone, 1986, with permission.)

BRAIN HEMORRHAGES: COMMON CLINICAL SYNDROMES

Location	Syndrome
Putaminal	Hemiparesis (smooth and steady onset); may progress to involve hemisensory loss, hemianopia, and aphasia (dominant hemisphere) or neglect (nondominant hemisphere); often associated with gaze deviation; syndrome may progress to coma and death
Thalamic	Initial deficit of hemisensory loss, later hemiparesis; with enlarging size, there may be vertical gaze palsy, retraction nystagmus, skew deviation, loss of convergence, ptosis and miosis, anisocoria, or unreactive pupils; if the hematoma is large, coma may be present from the onset; compression of CSF pathways may lead to hydrocephalus
Lobar	
Occipital	Pain about eye and dense hemianopsia
Temporal	Mild pain anterior to ear, aphasia (posterior), partial field defect
Frontal	Begins with severe arm weakness, minimal leg and face weakness, and frontal headache
Parietal	Anterior temporal headache, hemisensory deficit
Cerebellar	Sudden onset of nausea, vomiting, and inability to walk; also present may be headache, dizziness, impaired consciousness, appendicular hemorrhage, facial palsy, and ipsilateral gaze palsy
Pontine	Rapid onset of quadriplegia, decerebrate posturing, pinpoint pupils, oculomotor disturbances, and coma

(From Ojemann RG, Heros RC: Spontaneous brain hemorrhage. Stroke 14:468–475, 1983, with permission.)

CAUSES OF INTRACEREBRAL HEMORRHAGE

I. Hypertension
    A. Chronic effects of hypertension
    B. Malignant hypertension/hypertensive encephalopathy
II. Drugs
    A. Cocaine
    B. Pseudoephedrine
    C. Amphetamine
III. Vascular abnormalities
    A. Saccular aneurysm
    B. Arteriovenous malformations
    C. Angiomas
    D. Mycotic aneurysm
IV. Abnormal arteries
    A. Amyloid angiopathy
    B. Arteritis
V. Bleeding diatheses
    A. Anticoagulants
    B. Fibrinolytic agents
    C. Blood dyscrasias/coagulation disorders
VI. Head trauma
VII. Bleeding into preexisting lesions
    A. Tumors (primary or metastatic)
    B. Granulomas
    C. Meningitis
    D. Ischemic stroke with hemorrhagic conversion
    E. Abscess
VIII. Spontaneous

COMMON PRESENTING SYMPTOMS OF
SUBARACHNOID HEMORRHAGE

    I. Headache
    II. Nausea
    III. Vomiting
    IV. Brief loss of consciousness
    V. Neck stiffness or pain
    VI. Hemiparesis
    VII. Vertigo
    VIII. Faintness
    IX. Confusion
    X. Convulsions
    XI. Coma
    XII. Hearing loss
    XIII. Visual loss
    XIV. Diplopia
    XV. Malaise and diffuse aches
    XVI. Photophobia
    XVII. Back pain
    XVIII. Leg pain
    XIX. Ataxia
    XX. Speech disturbance
    XXI. Chest pain
    XXII. Paraparesis

(From Adams HP, et al: Pitfalls in the recognition of subarachnoid hemorrhage. JAMA 244:794, 1980, with permission.)

CLASSIFICATION OF PATIENTS
WITH INTRACRANIAL ANEURYSMS ACCORDING
TO SURGICAL RISK

Grade Category*	Criteria
I	Asymptomatic or minimal headache, slight nuchal rigidity
II	Moderate to severe headache, nuchal rigidity, no neurological deficit other than cranial nerve palsy
III	Drowsiness, confusion, or mild focal deficit
IV	Stupor, moderate to severe hemiparesis, possible early decerebrate rigidity, vegetative disturbances
V	Deep coma, decerebrate rigidity, moribund appearance

* Serious systemic disease (such as hypertension, diabetes mellitus, severe atherosclerosis, chronic pulmonary disease, and severe vasospasm seen on arteriography) results in placement of patient in the next higher category.
(From Report of the WHO Task Force on Stroke and Other Cerebrovascular Disorders: Stroke—1989: recommendations on stroke prevention, diagnosis, and therapy. Stroke 20:1407–1431, 1989, with permission.)

CAUSES OF DETERIORATION AFTER STROKE

I. Brain
- A. Cytotoxic edema
  1. → Herniation, vascular compression
- B. Recurrent stroke
  1. Embolism
  2. Progressive thrombosis
  3. Hypoperfusion
- C. Fluctuation of original deficit
- D. Hemorrhagic conversion
- E. Seizures
- F. Syndrome of inappropriate ADH secretion

II. Systemic factors
- A. Cardiac
  1. Arrhythmia
  2. Myocardial infarction
  3. Congestive heart failure
- B. Pulmonary
  1. Aspiration pneumonia
  2. Pulmonary embolism
- C. Septicemia (most commonly from pneumonia or UTI)
- D. Bed sores
- E. Peripheral nerve compression
- F. Muscle disuse atrophy
- G. Frozen joints
- H. Metabolic
  1. Electrolyte abnormalities
  2. Hypoglycemia

CNS VASCULITIS

I. Primary vasculitis
   A. Granulomatous angiitis of the nervous system (GANS)
   B. Cogan syndrome
   C. Eales disease
   D. Isolated spinal cord arteritis
II. Systemic vasculitis
   A. Giant cell (temporal) arteritis
   B. Polyarteritis nodosa group (always with systemic disease)
      1. Polyarteritis nodosa
      2. Churg-Strauss vasculitis
      3. "Amphetamine" vasculitis
      4. Hepatitis B
   C. Takayasu's arteritis
   D. Wegener's granulomatosis
   E. Lymphomatoid granulomatosis
   F. Henoch-Schönlein purpura
   G. Cryoglobulinemia
   H. Malignant angioendotheliomatosis
III. Connective tissue disease
   A. Lupus
   B. Progressive systemic sclerosis
   C. Mixed connective tissue disease
   D. Sjögren syndrome
   E. Rheumatoid disease
   F. Juvenile rheumatoid arthritis
   G. Polymyositis/dermatomyositis
   H. Behçet syndrome
IV. Miscellaneous
   A. Infectious
      1. TB
      2. Sarcoid
      3. Syphilis
      4. Lyme disease
      5. Mucormycosis
      6. Herpes zoster ophthalmicus angiitis
      7. Malaria

List Continues

CNS VASCULITIS (*Continued*)

B. Thrombotic thrombocytopenic purpura
C. Left atrial myxoma
D. Multiple cholesterol emboli
E. Inflammatory bowel disease

(Modified from Sigal LH: The neurologic presentation of vasculitic and rheumatologic syndromes. Medicine (Baltimore) 66:157–180, 1987, with permission.)

NIH STROKE SCALE*

Level of consciousness
    Alert   0
    Drowsy (arousable with mild stimulation)   1
    Lethargic (requires repeated or strong stimulation)   2
    Reflexive movements/no response   3

Level of consciousness questions (name month and age)
    Both correct   0
    One correct   1
    None correct   2

Level of consciousness commands (following commands)
    Obeys both correctly   0
    Obeys one correctly   1
    Both incorrect   2

Visual fields (to confrontation)
    No visual loss   0
    Partial hemianopia   1
    Complete hemianopia   2

Facial palsy
    None   0
    Minor   1
    Partial   2
    Complete   3

Motor: arm (examine 90° sitting or 45° if prone)
    Holds for 10 s   0
    Drifts before 10 s   1
    Some effort against gravity   2
    No effort   3

Motor: leg (supine-hold leg at 30°)
    Holds leg up for 5 s   0
    Falls to intermediate position before 5 s   1
    Falls to bed by 5 s   2
    No effort against   3

Limb ataxia
    None   0
    Present in one limb   1
    Present in two limbs   2

* A higher score signifies a worse clinical state.

List Continues

NIH STROKE SCALE* (*Continued*)

Sensory (pinprick)

Normal	0
Mild loss	1
Severe to total loss	2

Neglect

None	0
Visual, tactile, or auditory hemi-inattention	1
Profound hemi-inattention or >1 modality	2

Dysarthria

None	0
Mild to moderate (slurs, but understood)	1
Severe (unintelligible at times)	2

Language

Normal	0
Mild (dysnomia, paraphasias, mild aphasia)	1
Fully developed aphasic syndrome	2
Mute or global aphasia	3

(From Goldstein LB, Bertels C, Davis DN: Interrater reliability of the NIH stroke scale. Arch Neurol 46:660–662, 1989, with permission.)

Movement Disorders

See additional lists on pages 104–118.

NEUROLEPTIC-INDUCED MOVEMENT DISORDERS

  I. Early (hours, days)
- A. Acute dystonic reaction
- B. Acute dyskinesias
- C. Akathisia
- D. Malignant neuroleptic syndrome

 II. Intermediate (weeks, months)
- A. Parkinsonism (rigidity, tremor, bradykinesia, rabbit syndrome)

III. Late (years)
- A. Tardive dyskinesia (buccal-lingual-masticatory syndrome)
- B. Tardive dystonia
- C. Withdrawal emergent syndrome
- D. Tardive akathisia
- E. Tardive Tourette syndrome

MOST FREQUENT DIAGNOSES IN GAIT DISORDERS

I. Neurological
  A. Central
    1. Stroke
    2. Parkinsonism (see list of akinetic-rigid syndromes)
    3. Dementia
    4. Fear of falling
  B. Peripherala neuropathy
    1. Diabetes mellitus
    2. Alcoholism
    3. Vitamin B_{12} deficiency
  C. Eye and ear
    1. Presbyopia
    2. Cataracts
    3. Benign positional vertigo
    4. Menière's disease
    5. Multiple sensory deficit syndrome
  D. Unknown etiology
    1. Idiopathic gait disorder
II. Cardiovascular
  A. Heart
    1. Atherosclerotic heart disease, class II or greater
  B. Arterial
    1. Intermittent claudication
    2. Orthostatic hypotension
    3. Vertebrobasilar insufficiency
  C. Venous
    1. Chronic leg edema

MOST FREQUENT DIAGNOSES IN GAIT DISORDERS
(*Continued*)

III. Arthritic/musculoskeletal
- A. Joints
    1. Degenerative joint disease
    2. Disc disease
    3. Rheumatic arthritis
    4. Gout
    5. Cervical spondylosis
    6. Congenital or acquired deformity
- B. Bone
    1. Osteoporosis
    2. Paget's disease
- C. Muscles
    1. Thyroid disease
    2. Immobility
    3. Polymyalgia

(From Hough JC, McHenry MP, Kammer LM: Gait disorders in the elderly. Am Fam Phys 35:191–196, 1987, with permission.)

CONDITIONS ASSOCIATED WITH
BLEPHAROSPASM

    I. Reflex blepharospasm
    II. Essential blepharospasm
    III. Meigs syndrome
    IV. Tardive dyskinesia and dystonia
    V. Parkinson's disease
    VI. Huntington's disease
    VII. Wilson's disease
    VIII. Encephalitis
    IX. Midbrain infarction or demyelination
    X. Drugs
        A. Antipsychotics
        B. Antiemetics
        C. Anorectics
        D. Nasal decongestants
        E. L-dopa
    XI. Habit spasms
    XII. Tics (e.g., Gilles de la Tourette syndrome)
    XIII. Hemifacial spasm
    XIV. Facial nerve misdirection (e.g., aberrant regeneration)
    XV. Myokymia
    XVI. Myotonia
    XVII. Tetany
    XVIII. Tetanus
    XIX. Schwartz-Jampel syndrome
    XX. Ocular disease
    XXI. Seizures (absence, partial)
    XXII. Functional (hysterical)

(From Jankovic J, Havins WE, Wilkins RB: Blinking and blepharospasm. JAMA 248:3160–3164, 1982, with permission.)

Psychiatry and Behavioral Neurology

FEATURES THAT HELP DISTINGUISH DEPRESSION FROM DEMENTIA

Primary Depression	Primary Dementia
General	
Family usually aware of illness	Family unaware of illness
Onset dated and more acute	Insidious onset, broadly and vaguely dated
Symptoms of short duration	Symptoms of long duration
Rapid progression	Slow progression
Family history of affective disorder	Possible family history of Alzheimer's disease
Personal History	
Patient with history of depression	No history of depression
Patient complains of cognitive deficits and seeks help	No complaints of cognitive deficits
Patient complains in detail	Complaints are vague
Patient's complaints of cognitive deficits are emphasized	Deficit is concealed
Patient highlights his or her failures	Patient delights in his or her accomplishments
Patient makes little effort at task	Patient struggles with task
Patient does not try to keep up	Patient relies on notes, calendars, and the like
Patient is in distress	Patient is unconcerned
Affective symptoms pervasive	Affect is labile and shallow
Behavior incongruent with dysfunction	Behavior compatible with cognitive dysfunction
Examination	
No sun-downing	Sun-downs
Attention and concentration preserved	Faulty attention and concentration
"I don't know" answers are typical	Frequent "near miss" answers
"Don't know" answers on orientation	Orientation tests poor
Recent and remote memory loss are similar	Recent memory loss greater than remote memory loss
Decreased memory for specific periods is common	No gaps in memory
No glabellar or snout reflexes	Glabellar and snout reflexes present

List Continues

FEATURES THAT HELP DISTINGUISH
DEPRESSION FROM DEMENTIA (*Continued*)

Psychological Testing

Variable performance	Consistently poor performance
Weschler scale shows no typical pattern	Greater discrepancy between verbal and performance scores

Examination of Mental Status

No apraxia or agnosia	Has apraxia or agnosia
Will correct any word intrusions	Demonstrates word intrusions

Neurological Testing

CT scan normal	May see increased ventricular size and cortical atrophy on CT
Dexamethasone suppression test (DST) nonsuppressed (60%)	DST may or may not suppress

(From Winstead DK, Mielke DH: Different diagnosis between dementia and depression in the elderly. Neurol Clin 2:23–35, 1984, with permission.)

HACHINSKI ISCHEMIC SCORE FOR DEMENTIA*

Feature	Score
Abrupt onset	2
Stepwise deterioration	1
Fluctuating course	1
Nocturnal confusion	1
Relative preservation of personality	1
Depression	1
Somatic complaints	1
Emotional incontinence	1
History of hypertension	1
History of strokes	2
Evidence of associated atherosclerosis	1
Focal neurological symptoms	2
Focal neurological signs	2

* A score of ≥7 suggests multi-infarct dementia or a vascular component to the dementia.
(From Hachinski VC, et al: Cerebral blood flow in dementia. Arch Neurol 32:634, 1975, with permission.)

DRUGS THAT MAY INDUCE PARANOID OR SCHIZOPHRENIC-LIKE PSYCHOSES

I. Hallucinogens
  A. Lysergic acid (LSD)
  B. Mescaline
  C. Phencyclidine
  D. Dimethoxymethylamphetamine
II. CNS stimulants
  A. Amphetamines
  B. Cocaine
  C. Diethylpropion
  D. Phenmetrazine
  E. Ephedrine
  F. Pseudoephedrine
  G. Propylhexedrine
III. CNS depressants
  A. Ethyl alcohol
  B. Barbiturates
  C. Bromides
  D. Chloral hydrate
  E. Antihistamines
  F. Anticonvulsants (phenytoin, sulthiamine, ethosuximide)
IV. Antimicrobial drugs
  A. Isoniazid
  B. Cycloserine
  C. Ethionamide
  D. Atabrine
  E. Mepacrine
  F. Chloroquine
V. Cardiovascular drugs
  A. Digitalis
  B. Hydralazine
  C. Disopyramide
  D. Methyldopa
VI. Antiparkinsonian drugs
  A. Benzhexol
  B. Benztropine
  C. L-dopa
  D. Bromocriptine
VII. Miscellaneous drugs
  A. Corticosteroids
  B. ACTH

List Continues

DRUGS THAT MAY INDUCE PARANOID OR
SCHIZOPHRENIC-LIKE PSYCHOSES (*Continued*)

C. Indomethacin
D. Disulfiram
E. Dextropropoxyphene
F. Tocainide

(From Mastaglia FL: Iatrogenic (drug-induced) disorders of the nervous system. pp. 505–532. In Aminoff MJ (ed): Neurology and General Medicine. Churchill Livingstone, New York, 1989, with permission.)

Epilepsy and Seizures

CLASSIFICATION OF EPILEPSY

I. Partial
  A. Simple
    1. Motor
      a. Focal motor
      b. Focal motor with march (Jacksonian)
      c. Versive
      d. Postural
      e. Phonatory (e.g., vocalization or speech arrest)
    2. Sensory
      a. Somatosensory
      b. Visual
      c. Auditory
      d. Olfactory
      e. Gustatory
      f. Vertiginous
    3. Autonomic
      a. Epigastric sensation
      b. Pallor
      c. Sweating
      d. Flushing
      e. Piloerection
      f. Pupillary dilation
    4. Psychic
      a. Aphasic
      b. Dysmnestic (e.g., déjà vu)
      c. Cognitive (e.g., disorder of time sense)
      d. Affective (e.g., fear, anger)
      e. Illusions (e.g., macropsia, micropsia)
      f. Complex hallucinations (e.g., music, visual scenes)
  B. Complex
    1. Without impaired consciousness from start, beginning as simple partial
    2. With impaired consciousness from start
      a. Without automatisms
      b. With automatisms
  C. Secondarily generalized
    1. Secondary to complex partial
    3. Miscellaneous (may generalize to other than tonic-clonic seizure)
      a. West syndrome
      b. Lennox-Gastaut syndrome
      c. Progressive myoclonus epilepsies (see separate classification)

List Continues

CLASSIFICATION OF EPILEPSY (*Continued*)

II. Generalized
   A. Absence
      1. Classic absence with 3 Hz spike-and-wave
      2. Absence of juvenile myoclonic epilepsy
      3. Juvenile absence with diffuse 8–12 Hz rhythms
      4. Myoclonic absence with diffuse 3–6 Hz multi-spike-and-wave
      5. Myoclonic absence with automatisms and 12 Hz rhythm
   B. Tonic
   C. Clonic
   D. Tonic-clonic
   E. Myoclonic
      1. Myoclonic seizures of childhood
      2. Juvenile myoclonic seizures of Janz
   F. Akinetic
   G. Infantile spasms without West syndrome
III. Unclassified

PROGRESSIVE MYOCLONUS EPILEPSY (PME)

Common features are seizures (usually myoclonic, also tonic-clonic or others), progressive deficits (especially ataxia, dementia), familial
- I. Baltic myoclonus (Unverricht-Lundborg syndrome)
- II. Lafora body disease
- III. Lysosomal storage diseases
  - A. Neuronal ceroid-lipofuscinosis
    1. Late infantile neuronal-ceroid lipofuscinosis (Jansky-Biel-schowsky disease)
    2. Juvenile neuronal ceroid-lipofuscinosis (Spielmeyer-Vogt or Batten's disease)
    3. Adult neuronal ceroid-lipofuscinosis (Kufs disease)
  - B. Sialidoses
    1. Cherry-red spot myoclonus syndrome (type I)
    2. Type II
  - C. GM_2 gangliosidosis
  - D. Gaucher's disease
- IV. Biotin deficiency
- V. Mitochondrial encephalomyopathy
  - A. MERRF
  - B. PME and deafness (May-White syndrome)
  - C. PME and lipomas (Ekbom syndrome)
- VI. Action myoclonus/renal failure syndrome
- VII. Hallervorden-Spatz disease
- VIII. Juvenile neuroaxonal dystrophy
- IX. Dentato-rubro-pallido-luysian atrophy
- X. Intraneuronal inclusion disease

(From Berkovic SF, Andermann F, Carpenter S et al: Progressive myoclonus epilepsies: specific causes and diagnosis. N Engl J Med 315:296–305, 1986, with permission.)

CAUSES OF SEIZURES BY AGE

I. Newborn
  A. Perinatal hypoxia and ischemia
  B. Drug withdrawal
  C. Hypocalcemia
  D. Hypomagnesemia
  E. Hyperbilirubinemia (kernicterus)
  F. Hypoglycemia
  G. Water intoxication
  H. Intracranial hemorrhage
   I. Intracranial birth injury
  J. Inborn errors of metabolism
  K. Pyridoxine deficiency
  L. Congenital malformations of brain
  M. Intracranial infection
  N. Sepsis
II. Infancy
  A. Congenital defects
  B. Inborn errors of metabolism
  C. Idiopathic
  D. Acute infection
  E. Trauma
  F. Febrile convulsions

CAUSES OF SEIZURES BY AGE (*Continued*)

III. Childhood
    A. Trauma
    B. Congenital defects
    C. Arteriovenous malformation
    D. CNS infection
IV. Adolescent/young adult
    A. Idiopathic
    B. Trauma
    C. Drug, alcohol withdrawal
    D. Arteriovenous malformation
    E. Brain tumor
 V. Older adults
    A. Alcoholism
    B. Brain tumor
    C. Cerebrovascular disease
    D. Trauma
    E. Metabolic disorders
    F. Uremia
    G. Hepatic failure
    H. Electrolyte abnormalities
    I. Hypoglycemia
    J. CNS infection

DRUGS REPORTED TO CAUSE SEIZURES

I. Antidepressants
   A. Imipramine
   B. Amitriptyline
   C. Doxepin
   D. Nortriptyline
   E. Maprotiline
   F. Mianserin
   G. Nomifensine
   H. Bupropion

II. Antipsychotics
   A. Chlorpromazine
   B. Thioridazine
   C. Perphenazine
   D. Trifluoperazine
   D. Prochlorperazine
   F. Haloperidol

III. Analgesics
   A. Fentanyl
   B. Meperidine
   C. Pentazocine
   D. Propoxyphene
   E. Cocaine
   F. Mefenamic acid

IV. Local anesthetics
   A. Lidocaine
   B. Mepivacaine
   C. Procaine
   D. Bupivacaine
   E. Etidocaine

V. General anesthetics
   A. Ketamine
   B. Halothane
   C. Althesin
   D. Enflurane
   E. Propanidid
   F. Methohexital

VI. Antimicrobials
   A. Penicillin
   B. Synthetic penicillins (oxacillin, carbenicillin, ticarcillin)
   C. Ampicillin
   D. Cephalosporins

DRUGS REPORTED TO CAUSE SEIZURES (*Continued*)

    E. Metronidazole
    F. Nalidixic acid
    G. Isoniazid
    H. Cycloserine
    I. Pyrimethamine
VII. Antineoplastics
    A. Chlorambucil
    B. Vincristine
    C. Methotrexate
    D. Cytosine
    E. Arabinoside
    F. Misonidazole
    G. BCNU
    H. PALA
VIII. Bronchodilators
    A. Aminophylline
    B. Theophylline
  IX. Sympathomimetics
    A. Ephedrine
    B. Terbutaline
    C. Phenylpropanolamine
  X. Others
    A. Insulin
    B. Antihistamines
    C. Anticholinergics
    D. Baclofen
    E. Cyclosporin A
    F. Lithium
    G. Atenolol
    H. Disopyramide
    I. Phencyclidine
    J. Amphetamines
    K. Domperidone
    L. Doxapram
    M. Ergonovine
    N. Folic acid
    O. Camphor
    P. Methylxanthenes
    Q. TRH
    R. Vitamin K oxide
    S. Aqueous iodinated contrast media

List Continues

DRUGS REPORTED TO CAUSE SEIZURES (*Continued*)

    T. Oxytocin
    U. Hyperosmolar parenteral solutions
    V. Hyperbaric oxygen
    W. Anticonvulsants
    X. Methylphenidate

(From Mastaglia FL: Iatrogenic (drug-induced) disorders of the nervous system. pp. 505–532. In Aminoff MJ (ed.): Neurology and General Medicine. Churchill Livingstone, New York, 1989, with permission.)

RELATIVE EPILEPTOGENIC POTENCY OF VARIOUS GROUPS OF PSYCHOTROPIC DRUGS

Psychotropic Drug	Relative Epileptogenic Potency
Neuroleptics	
Phenothiazines	
Chlorpromazine	Marked
Promazine HCl	Marked
Thioridazine	Slight
Mesoridazine	Slight
Perphenazine	Moderate
Fluphenazine	Slight
Thioxanthenes	
Thiothixene	Moderate
Butyrophenones	
Haloperidol	Moderate
Indole derivatives	
Molindone HCl	Slight
Antidepressants	
Tricyclics	
Imipramine HCl	Slight
Amitriptyline HCl	Moderate
Monoamine oxidase inhibitors	
Nialamide	Slight
Inorganic salts	
Lithium carbonate	Marked
Anxiolytics	
Meprobamate	Doubtful
Chlordiazepoxide	None (except on discontinuation)
Diazepam	None (except on discontinuation)
Psychostimulants	
Methylphenidate HCl	Slight
Dextroamphetamine	Doubtful

(From Itil TM, Soldatos C: Epileptogenic side effects of psychotropic drugs. JAMA 244:1460–1463, 1980, with permission.)

CONDITIONS THAT MAY MIMIC SEIZURES

   I. Hypoglycemia
  II. Syncope
 III. Hyperventilation
  IV. Cardiac arrhythmia
   V. Migraine
  VI. Stroke/TIA
 VII. Breath-holding spell
VIII. Episodic movement disorder
  IX. Metabolic encephalopathy (asterixis and change in mentation)
   X. Functional episode

COMMON ANTICONVULSANT MEDICATIONS

Drug	Dose (mg)	Half-life (hrs)	Therapeutic Level (μg/ml)	Toxicity	Effects of Other Medications on Drug Levels
Phenytoin	300–400	24±12	10–20	Dose related: nystagmus, ataxia, drowsiness, cognitive impairment, dyskinesias. Not dose related: blood dyscrasias, gingival hyperplasia, Stevens-Johnson syndrome, osteopenia, folate deficiency, hepatic failure, lymphadenopathy, neuropathy.	Carbamazepine increases, occasionally decreases; phenobarbital, no change; valproate decreases.
Phenobarbital	20–120	96±12	15–35	Dose related: sedation, ataxia, hyperactivity, cognitive impairment. Not dose related: blood dyscrasias, skin rash, osteopenia, allergic dermatitis, hepatic failure.	Carbamazepine, no change; phenytoin increases; valproate increases.
Ethosuximide	750–1,000	60±10	40–100	Hiccups, GI distress, drowsiness, ataxia, blood dyscrasias, skin rash, dizziness.	
Carbamazepine	800–1,600	16±6	8–12	Dose related: visual changes, drowsiness, ataxia, cognitive impairment, dyskinesia, cardiac conduction abnormalities, vertigo, dry mouth. Not dose related: Stevens-Johnson syndrome, hepatic failure, renal failure, GI distress, blood dyscraias.	Phenobarbital decreases; phenytoin decreases.
Sodium valproate	750–1,500	12±6	50–100	Dose related: GI distress, tremor, behavioral changes. Not dose related: hair loss, weight gain, nausea, liver toxicity, leukopenia, pancreatitis.	Carbamazepine decreases; phenobarbital decreases; phenytoin decreases.
Clonazepam	1–10	36±12	10–70	Ataxia, drowsiness, behavioral disturbances, slurred speech, dysarthria, blood dyscrasias.	

DRUGS USED IN DIFFERENT SEIZURE TYPES

I. Partial seizures
  A. Carbamazepine
  B. Phenytoin
  C. Phenobarbital
  D. Clonazepam
  E. Valproate
II. Generalized seizures
  A. Tonic, clonic, and tonic-clonic
      1. Carbamazepine
      2. Phenytoin
      3. Valproate
      4. Phenobarbital
      5. Clonazepam
  B. Absence
      1. Valproate
      2. Ethosuximide
      3. Clonazepam
  C. Myoclonic
      1. Infancy
          a. ACTH
          b. Steroids
          c. Phenobarbital
          d. Valproate
          e. Clonazepam
          f. Nitrazepam
      2. Childhood
          a. Phenobarbital
          b. Valproate
          c. Clonazepam
          d. Nitrazepam
      3. Adolescence
          a. Clonazepam
          b. Valproate

(Modified from Eadie MJ, Tyrer JH: Anticonvulsant Therapy: Pharmacological Basis and Practice. Churchill Livingstone, New York, 1989, with permission.)

PREGNANCY AND ANTICONVULSANTS

Drug	Steady-state Levels	Absorption	Distribution to Fetus	Metabolism	Binding
Phenytoin	Decrease by 50–100%	Marked decrease in rare cases	Rapid	Increased	Decreased
Carbamazepine	Decrease by 25–50%	Probably not altered	Rapid	Increased	No significant change
Valproate	Some decrease	Not altered	Rapid	Increased	Decreased
Phenobarbital and primidone	Some decrease	Not altered	Rapid	Increased	No significant change

(From Leppik IE, Rask CA: Pharmacokinetics of antiepileptic drugs during pregnancy. Semin Neurol 8:240–246, 1988, with permission.)

CONGENITAL DEFECTS POSSIBLY ASSOCIATED WITH ANTICONVULSANTS

I. Phenytoin and hydantoins
   A. Cleft lip and palate
   B. Ectrodactyly (congenital absence of all or part of a digit)
   C. Hydronephrosis
   D. Hydrocephalus
   E. Peritoneal and renal hemorrhage
   F. Decreased growth of long bones
   G. Congenital heart malformations
   H. Alimentary abnormalities

II. Carbamazepine
   A. ?Fetal head growth retardation

III. Barbiturate and related anticonvulsants
   A. Cleft lip
   B. Cleft palate
   C. Blood coagulation defects

IV. Succinimides
   A. Little work done since the indication for the use of ethosuximide (absence seizures) usually ceases before the usual age of reproduction.

V. Troxidone
   A. Low-set ears
   B. Palatal abnormalities
   C. Irregular teeth
   D. V-shaped eyebrows
   E. Altered speech

VI. Benzodiazepine
   A. ?Cleft palate
   B. ?Cleft lip

VII. Valproate
   A. Spina bifida

VIII. Chlormethiazole
   A. No clear associations

(Modified from Eadie MJ, Tyrer JH: Anticonvulsant Therapy: Pharmacological Basis and Practice. Churchill Livingstone, New York, 1989, with permission.)

Spinal Cord Lesions

LOW BACK PAIN

I. Local structural disease
   - A. Herniated nucleus pulposus
   - B. Spondylosis (osteoarthritis)
   - C. Spinal stenosis
   - D. Scoliosis
   - E. Osteoporosis
   - F. Myofascial syndromes ("fibrositis")
   - G. Neoplastic (primary or secondary; epidural, intradural, intramedullary; meningeal carcinomatosis)

II. Retroperitoneal disease
   - A. Aortic aneurysm
   - B. Neoplasm
   - C. Renal disease
   - D. Penetrating ulcer
   - E. Pancreatitis

III. Metabolic
   - A. Diabetic neuropathy
   - B. Gout
   - C. Paget's disease

IV. Infection
   - A. Infection of disc/vertebra
   - B. Epidural abscess
   - C. Meningitis
   - D. Herpes zoster

V. Inflammatory
   - A. Rheumatoid arthritis
   - B. Ankylosing spondylitis
   - C. Reiter syndrome
   - D. Psoriatic arthritis
   - E. Arachnoiditis

VI. Trauma
   - A. Musculoligamentous sprain/strain
   - B. Spondylolysis/spondylolisthesis

VII. Psychogenic
   - A. Chronic pain syndrome
   - B. Malingering
   - C. Substance abuse

SPINAL ARTERY SYNDROMES

I. Anterior spinal artery syndrome
    A. Radicular and ascending leg pain
    B. Sudden nonprogressive paraplegia
    C. Flaccid legs, which soon become spastic
    D. Areflexia, which becomes hyperreflexia with Babinski sign
    E. Sensory level for pain and temperature
    F. Preservation of touch, position, and vibration sense
    G. Urinary and fecal incontinence (rare)
    H. Later focal atrophy and wasting (with cervical or lumbar infarction)
II. Posterior spinal artery syndrome
    A. Suspended global anesthesia
    B. Local tendon and cutaneous reflex loss
    D. Dorsal column sensory loss and level
    D. Anterior cord spared

(From Buchan AM, Barnett HJM: Infarction of the spinal cord. pp. 707–719. In: Stroke. Churchill Livingstone, New York, 1986, with permission.)

LUMBAR STENOSIS (SIGNS AND SYMPTOMS)

Symptom or Sign	Prevalence (%)
Pseudoclaudication*	94
Standing discomfort	94
Description	
Pain	93
Numbness	63
Weakness	43
Bilateral	69
Site	
Whole limb	78
Above knee alone	15
Below knee alone	7
Radicular pain only	6
Ankle reflex decreased or absent	43
Knee reflex decreased or absent	18
Objective weakness	37
Positive straight leg raising	10

* Pseudoclaudication is defined as discomfort in the buttock(s), thigh(s), or leg(s) on standing or walking, relieved by rest (lying, sitting, or flexion at the waist).

(From Hall S, Bartleson JD, Onofrio BM, et al: Lumbar spinal stenosis. Ann Intern Med 103:271–275, 1985, with permission.)

NONSTRUCTURAL CAUSES OF ACUTE TRANSVERSE MYELITIS

I. Infection
  A. Bacterial
    1. Syphilis
    2. Mycoplasma
    3. Parasitic
    4. Schistosomiasis
    5. Cat-stratch fever
    6. Tetanus
    7. Tuberculosis
  B. Viral
    1. Mumps
    2. Measles
    3. Rubella
    4. Influenza
    5. Herpes zoster and simplex
    6. CMV
    7. Hepatitis A and B
    8. Poliomyelitis and other enteroviruses
    9. HIV
    10. Rabies
  C. Lyme disease
  D. Larva migrans
II. Myelin
  A. Multiple sclerosis (Devic's disease)
  B. Postinfectious

NONSTRUCTURAL CAUSES OF ACUTE TRANSVERSE MYELITIS (*Continued*)

III. Vascular/Inflammatory
   - A. Infarct
   - B. AVM
   - C. Granulomatous disease (sarcoidosis)
   - D. Sjögren syndrome
   - E. Systemic lupus
   - F. Rheumatoid arthritis
   - G. Mixed connective tissue diseases
IV. Metabolic
   - A. Endotoxemia
   - B. Heroin
   - C. Intra-arterial or IM penicillin
   - D. Arsenicals
   - E. Sulfas
   - F. Benzene
   - G. Heavy metals
 V. Trauma
   - A. Radiation therapy

CAUSES OF SPINAL CORD INFARCTION

	Ischemic	**Emboli**
Heart	Hypotension Cardiac arrest	Subacute bacterial endocarditis Atrial myxoma
Aorta	Atherosclerosis Aortic surgery (with clamping) Dissecting aneurysm Coarctation of aorta	Aortic angiography Cholesterol emboli Saddle emboli Aortic trauma Intra-aortic balloon pump counterpulsation
Vertebra	Vertebral occlusion Vertebral dissection Sickle cell anemia Fracture and spinal dislocations	Vertebral angiography
Intercostal arteries	Thoracoplasty Coarctation operation	
Radicular arteries	Arteriosclerosis Ligation during surgery Cervical spondylosis Cervical sprain Caisson disease Plasmacytoma Reticulum cell sarcoma Lumbar sympathectomy Aneurysm artery of Adamkiewicz	Aortic emboli Spinal angiography

CAUSES OF SPINAL CORD INFARCTION (*Continued*)

	Ischemic	**Emboli**
Anterior median spinal artery	Atherosclerosis Diabetes Syphilis Cervical disc	Aortic embolization
Sulcal arteries	Hypertensive lacuna disease Diabetes Polyarteritis nodosa Infection, TB, syphilis	Aortic embolization Renal embolization
Pial microcirculation	In association with AVM Adhesive arachnoiditis Neoplastic spread Subarachnoid hemor-rhage Infective and granulo-matous meningitis	? Emboli from AVM

(From Buchan AM, Barnett HJM: Infarction of the spinal cord. pp. 707–719. In: Churchill Livingstone, New York, 1986, with permission.)

DISEASES THAT CAN MIMIC OR ARE ASSOCIATED WITH MOTOR NEURON DISEASE

   I. Multiple radiculopathies with cervical spondylitic myelopathy
  II. Syringomyelia
 III. Spinal AVM
  IV. Hyperparathyroidism
   V. Multiple myeloma
  VI. Macroglobulinemia
 VII. Hyperthyroidism
VIII. Familial ALS
  IX. Guamanian ALS/dementia/Parkinson's complex (2-Amino-3-(methylamino)-propanoic acid [BMAA] in cycad flour)
   X. Heavy metal intoxication
       A. Lead
       B. Mercury
  XI. Antibodies to GM_1 and GD_{1b} in patients with motor neuron disease without plasma cell dyscrasia
 XII. Antimyelin/DNA antibody
XIII. Antimyelin-associated glycoprotein
 XIV. Monoclonal IgMs with anti-Gal(beta 1-3) GalNAc activity
  XV. Syphilis
 XVI. Decrease/absence of hexosaminidase A activity
XVII. Konzo (upper motor neuron disease in Tanzania)
XVIII. HTLV-I–associated encephalomyelopathy
 XIX. Myokymia of the tongue in a case of brainstem tumor
  XX. Multifocal acquired demyelinating neuropathy
 XXI. Polio/postpolio syndrome
XXII. GM_1 gangliosidosis
XXIII. Debrancher enzyme deficiency

Neuromuscular Diseases

ACUTE GENERALIZED WEAKNESS

I. Motor neuron disorders
   A. Poliomyelitis
   B. Other enterovirus infections
   C. Paralytic (dumb) rabies
II. Polyneuropathy
   A. Guillain-Barré syndrome
   B. Hepatic porphyrias
   C. Diphtheria
   D. Arsenic poisoning
   E. Tick paralysis
   F. Podophyllum poisoning
   G. Acute hypophosphatemia
   H. Acute exacerbation of chronic hyperkalemia
   I. Shellfish and seafood poisoning
III. Disorders of neuromuscular transmission
   A. Myasthenia gravis
   B. Botulism
   C. Magnesium excess
   D. Drugs (trimethaphan, antibiotics)
   E. Neurotoxic snake bites
IV. Myopathy
   A. Acute hypokalemic paralysis
   B. Chronic potassium depletion
   C. Thyrotoxic periodic paralysis
   D. Familial hypokalemic periodic paralysis
   E. Acute hyperkalemic periodic paralysis
   F. Necrotic myopathies

(From Layzer RB: Diagnosis of neuromuscular disorders. p. 14. In Neuro-muscular Manifestations of Systemic Disease. FA Davis, Philadelphia, 1985, with permission.)

SUBACUTE AND CHRONIC GENERALIZED
WEAKNESS

 I. Endocrine disorders
   A. Hyperthyroidism
   B. Hypothyroidism
   C. Hyperadrenalism
   D. Nelson syndrome
   E. Acromegaly
   F. Vitamin D deficiency or resistance
   G. Hyperparathyroidism
 II. Degenerative
   A. Amyotrophic lateral sclerosis
   B. Motor neuron disorders
 III. Paraneoplastic
   A. Carcinomatous polioencephalomyelitis
   B. Subacute motor neuropathy in lymphoma
   C. Carcinomatous proximal neuromyopathy
   D. Carcinomatous myopathy
 IV. Polyneuropathies
 V. Disorders of neuromuscular transmission
   A. Myasthenia gravis
   B. Eaton-Lambert syndrome
   C. Drugs (beta-blockers, lithium)
 VI. Myopathy
   A. Mineral and electrolyte disorders
   B. Chronic potassium deficiency
   C. Polymyositis/dermatomyositis
   D. Chronic phosphorous deficiency
   E. Noninflammatory necrotic myopathy
 VII. Infectious disorders
   A. Toxoplasmosis
   B. Trichinosis
   C. Cysticercosis
   D. Sarcoidosis
 VIII. Amyloidosis
 IX. Drugs/toxins

SUBACUTE AND CHRONIC GENERALIZED
WEAKNESS (*Continued*)

A. Subacute and chronic alcoholic myopathy
B. Corticosteroids, rifampicin, colchicine
C. Clofibrate, drugs causing potassium deficiency, beta-blockers, emetine
D. Chloroquine

(From Layzer RB: Diagnosis of neuromuscular disorders. p. 14. In Neuromuscular Manifestations of Systemic Disease. FA Davis, Philadelphia, 1985, with permission.)

FASCICULATIONS*

    I. Benign fasciculations
   II. Fatigue
  III. Nerve terminal trauma and regeneration
  IV. Hypokalemia
   V. Hypocalcemia
  VI. Hyperthyroidism
 VII. Thyrotoxic myopathy
VIII. Cholinergic medications
  IX. Anterior horn cell diseases
     Q. Amyotrophic lateral sclerosis
     B. Polio
     C. Spinal cord injury
     D. Anterior spinal artery infarction
     E. Progressive spinal muscular atrophy
     F. Syringomyelia
     G. Intramedullary spinal tumors
     H. Cervical spondylosis
   X. Uremia
  XI. Carcinomatous neuropathy
 XII. Neuropathy associated with heavy metals (e.g., lead, mercury)

* Contractions of large groups of muscle fibers, usually supplied by a single anterior horn cell. May be seen through the skin as a small twitch.

FOCAL NEUROPATHIES

I. Trauma to nerve
   A. Transection
   B. Focal crush
   C. Stretch and traction
   D. Surgery
   E. Compression
   F. Birth trauma
   G. Entrapment
   H. Injections (antibiotics, addictive drugs, analeptics)
II. Infections (direct infection of nerve)
   A. Syphilis
   B. Tuberculosis
   C. Leprosy
   D. Herpes zoster
   E. Typhus
III. Toxins
   A. Lead (classically radial nerve)
   B. Tetanus antitoxin (most commonly brachial plexopathy)
   C. Insect stings (e.g., ticks, bees, wasps, ants, spiders)
IV. Vascular
   A. Small artery disease
      1. Arteritis (polyarteritis, rheumatoid arthritis)
      2. Diabetes
      3. Rheumatoid arthritis
      4. Amyloid
   B. Blood viscosity disorders (macroglobulinemia, cryogobulinemia, sickle cell disase, polycythemia, thrombocytopenia)
   C. Clotting abnormalities (hemophilia, anticoagulation)
   D. Large artery disease
      1. Emboli (cardiac, subacute bacterial endocarditis, tumor, air)
      2. Thromboangiitis obliterans (Buerger's disease)
      3. Thrombosis (arteriosclerotic occlusive disease)
V. Infiltration/compression
   A. Tumors
      1. Nerve fiber tumors (e.g., ganglioneuroma)
      2. Nerve sheath tumors (e.g., neurofibroma)
      3. Metastatic disease
      4. Lymphoma
      5. Leukemia
      6. Granuloma
      7. Sarcoid

FOCAL NEUROPATHIES (*Continued*)

   B. Amyloid
   C. Porphyria
   D. Immunological
       1. Brachial and lumbar plexopathy
VI. Miscellaneous
   A. Cold
       1. Trench foot
       2. Immersion foot

NEUROPATHIES THAT CAN PRESENT WITH PREDOMINANTLY MOTOR SYMPTOMS

   I. Guillain-Barré syndrome
   II. Motor neuropathy in lymphoma
   III. Infectious mononucleosis
   IV. Infectious hepatitis
   V. Toxic neuropathies
       A. Lead
       B. Mercury
       C. Nitrofurantoin
       D. Dapsone
   VI. Porphyria
   VII. Diabetic amyotrophy
   VIII. Hereditary sensorimotor neuropathy (types I and II)
   IX. Subacute paraneoplastic motor neuropathy

NEUROPATHIES THAT CAN PRESENT WITH PREDOMINANTLY SENSORY SYMPTOMS

    I. Diabetes
    II. Uremia
    III. Vitamin B_{12} deficiency
    IV. Amyloidosis
    V. Leprosy
    VI. Pyridoxine excess
    VII. AIDS-related sensory neuropathy
    VIII. Paraneoplastic sensory neuropathy
    IX. Hereditary sensory neuropathy (types I, II, III, IV)
    X. Tangier disease
    XI. Toxic
        A. Chloramphenicol
        B. Glutethimide
        C. Metronidazole
        D. Nitrous oxide
        E. Cisplatin
        F. Arsenic
        G. Thallium

NEUROPATHIES THAT CAN PRESENT WITH PREDOMINANTLY AUTONOMIC INVOLVEMENT

    I. Amyloidosis
   II. Diabetes
  III. Alcoholic neuropathy
  IV. Familial dysautonomias (Riley-Day syndrome, hereditary sensory neuropathy type III)
   V. Guillain-Barré syndrome
  VI. Acute intermittent porphyria
 VII. Chronic sensory and autonomic neuropathy
VIII. Other neuropathies associated with autonomic dysfunction, but usually not clinically important
     A. Toxic neuropathies (vincristine, acrylamide, heavy metals, organic solvents)
     B. HSM I, II, and V
     C. Malignancy
     D. Vitamin B_{12} deficiency
     E. Rheumatoid arthritis
     F. Chronic renal failure
     G. Systemic lupus erythematosis
     H. Mixed connective tissue disease
      I. Fabry's disease
      J. Chronic inflammatory polyneuropathy

(From McLeod JG, Tuck RR: Disorders of the autonomic nervous system. Ann Neurol 21:419–430, 1987, with permission.)

PAINFUL NEUROPATHIES

I. Diffuse
   A. Diabetes mellitus
   B. Alcoholic-nutritional
   C. Amyloid
   D. Fabry's disease
   E. Dominantly inherited sensory neuropathy
   F. AIDS-associated neuropathy
   G. Toxic
      1. Arsenic
      2. Thallium
      3. Chloramphenicol
      4. Metronidazole
   H. Guillain-Barré syndrome (transient muscle aching)
   I. Paraneoplastic sensory neuropathy
   J. Multiple myeloma
   K. Tangier disease
II. Focal
   A. Ischemic neuropathy
   B. Polyarteritis nodosa
   C. Diabetic mononeuropathy
   D. Diabetic amyotrophy
   E. Idiopathic brachial plexopathy
   F. Compressive neuropathies (carpal tunnel, meralgia paresthetica)
   G. Herpes zoster

POLYNEUROPATHIES CLASSIFIED ACCORDING TO TEMPORAL COURSE

I. Fulminating (hours)
   A. Food poisoning (e.g., shellfish)
   B. Acute hyperkalemia
   C. Acute hypophosphatemia
   D. Podophyllum poisoning
II. Acute (days)
   A. Guillain-Barré syndrome
   B. Porphyria
   C. Diphtheria
   D. Arsenic poisoning
   E. Tick paralysis
III. Subacute (weeks or months) (see separate list)
   A. Inflammatory
   B. Nutritional
   C. Toxic
   D. Metabolic
   E. Paraneoplastic
IV. Chronic (years)
   A. Chronic idiopathic polyneuritis
   B. Benign paraproteinemia
   C. Primary amyloidosis
   D. Diabetes mellitus
   E. Genetic/inherited diseases
V. Relapsing
   A. Idiopathic polyneuritis
   B. Benign paraproteinemia
   C. Collagen-vascular disorders
   D. Paraneoplastic
   E. Repeated toxin exposure
   F. Refsum's disease

(From Layzer RB: Diagnosis of neuromuscular disorders. p. 14. In Neuromuscular Manifestations of Systemic Disease. FA Davis, Philadelphia, 1985, with permission.)

CONDITIONS ASSOCIATED WITH CARPAL TUNNEL SYNDROME

    I. Spontaneous
    II. Trauma
    III. Occupational neuropathy
    IV. Pregnancy
    V. Degenerative joint disease
    VI. Rheumatoid arthritis
    VII. Diabetes mellitus
    VIII. Ganglion
    IX. Congenital abnormalities
    X. Myxedema
    XI. Acromegaly
    XII. Lupus erythematosis
    XIII. Scleroderma
    XIV. Gout
    XV. Leprosy
    XVI. Tuberculosis
    XVII. Pyogenic infections
    XVIII. Sarcoidosis
    XIX. Hereditary primary amyloidosis and multiple myeloma
    XX. Mucopolysaccharidosis
    XXI. Congestive heart failure
    XXII. Paget's disease
    XXIII. Forearm arteriovenous fistulas
    XXIV. Familial
    XXV. Benign tumors

(From Baker AB, Baker LH: Clinical Neurology. Vol. 4. JB Lippincott, Philadelphia, 1988, p. 42, with permission.)

DISEASES IN WHICH A NERVE BIOPSY MAY BE DIAGNOSTIC

Disease	Biopsy Findings
Leprosy	Inflammatory granuloma (may see central necrosis) with epithelioid cells, multinucleated giant cells, and lymphocytes; bacilli rarely seen; in lepromatous forms, there is Schwann cell colonization and invasion of macrophages by bacteria (lepra cells).
Amyloidosis	Demonstration of amyloid (lime-green fluorescence in polarized light after staining with Congo red).
Sarcoidosis	Granulomas without necrosis; segmental demyelination.
Metachromatic leukodystrophy	Reduction in myelinated fibers with segmental demyelination and remyelination leading to hypertrophy; characteristically there is accumulation of 1-μm metachromatic granules in the perinuclear region of the Schwann cell; stored sulfatide may be seen.
Krabbe's disease	Segmental demyelination with increased acid phosphatase activity.
Fabry's disease	There is a loss of small fibers and accumulation (lamellated inclusions) of ceramide trihexoside in the perineural cells and vascular endothelium.
Tangier disease	Accumulation of lipid droplets (neural lipids and cholesterol esters) in Schwann cells; loss of unmyelinated axons.
Hypertrophic neuropathies	Thickened and enlarged nerves (Schwann cell proliferation) are due to repeated demyelination and remyelination; seen in Charcot-Marie-Tooth disease, Dejerine-Sottas syndrome, Refsum's disease, neurofibromatosis, amyloidosis, leprosy, chronic demyelinative polyneuritis, and acromegaly.
Hereditary sensory motor neuropathies	Type I (Charcot-Marie-Tooth disease, hypertrophic form): reduced myelinated nerve fibers; hypertrophic changes from Schwann cell proliferation (from repeated segmental demyelination and remyelination). Type II (Charcot-Marie-Tooth disease, neuronal form): similar clinical picture of HSMN type I, but biopsy specimens show some axonal loss with little demyelination. Type III (Dejerine-Sottas syndrome): onion bulb formation with thinly myelinated fibers.
Toxic	*N*-hexane: axonal balloons; acrylamide: paranodal accumulation of neurofilaments with distal axonal degeneration; methylbutylketone: axonal balloons.
Giant axonal neuropathy	Segmental axonal dilatation packed with small neurofilaments.
Radiation injury	Axonal loss with extensive fibrosis.
Vasculitides (e.g., polyarteritis nodosa)	Multifocal necrotizing arteritis of the vasanervorum.

NEUROMUSCULAR JUNCTION DISEASES

   I. Myasthenia gravis
  II. Eaton-Lambert syndrome
 III. Botulism
 IV. Congenital myasthenias
  V. Snake envenomation (cobra, sea snake, coral snake, krait, mamba, viper, South American rattlesnake)
 VI. Arthropod envenomation (black widow, funnel-web spider, scorpion, tick paralysis)
VII. Drugs/toxins
   A. Antibiotics
     1. Streptomycin
     2. Gentamicin
     3. Neomycin
     4. Kanamycin
     5. Tobramycin
     6. Lincomycin
     7. Clindamycin
     8. Polymyxin B
     9. Tetracyclines
   10. Colistin
   11. Ampicillin
   B. Cardiac drugs
     1. Procainamide
     2. Quinidine
     3. Propranolol and other beta-blockers
     4. Bretylium
     5. Lidocaine
     6. Trimethaphan
     7. Calcium channel blockers

NEUROMUSCULAR JUNCTION DISEASES (*Continued*)

- C. Antirheumatic drugs
    1. Chloroquine
    2. D-penicillamine
- D. Psychotrophic drugs
    1. Phenelzine
    2. Lithium
    3. Chlorpromazine
- E. Anticonvulsants
    1. Phenytoin
    2. Trimethadione
- F. Anesthetics
    1. Curare and its derivatives
    2. Methoxyflurane
    3. Ether
    4. Procaine
    5. Lidocaine
- G. Hormones
    1. ACTH
    2. Corticosteroids
    3. Thyroid hormones
- H. Miscellaneous
    1. Magnesium
    2. Calcium
    3. Tetanus antitoxin
    4. Acetylcholinesterase inhibitors
    5. Any respiratory depressants
    6. Carnitine

COMMON MUSCULAR DYSTROPHIES

	Duchenne	**Facioscapulo-humeral**	**Limb-Girdle**	**Myotonic**
Sex	Male	Both	Both	Both
Onset	<5 yr	Adolescence	Adolescence	Infancy and adolescence
Initial symptoms	Pelvic	Shoulder-girdle	Either	Hands/feet
Face involved	No	Always	No	Often
Pseudohypertrophy	80%	No	Rare	No
Progression	Rapid	Slow	Slow	Slow
Inheritance	X-linked recessive	Autosomal dominant	Autosomal recessive	Autosomal dominant
Serum enzymes	Very high	Normal	Slightly increased	Normal
Myotonia	No	No	No	Yes

MISLEADING CAUSES OF ELEVATED SERUM CPK

I. Probably of muscle origin
   A. Trauma
   B. Surgery
   C. Severe burns
   D. Muscle hemorrhage
   E. Intramuscular injections
   F. Strenuous exercise
   G. Involuntary spasms or rigidity
   H. Hypothermia
   I. Hyperthermia
   J. Alcoholism
   K. Electric shock, lightning stroke
   L. Large muscle mass
   M. Malignant hyperthermia trait
   N. Chronic idiopathic CPK elevation

II. CNS disease
   A. Stroke
   B. Subarachnoid hemorrhage
   C. Bacterial meningitis
   D. Head injury

III. Cardiac injury
   A. Acute myocardial infarction
   B. Electrical cardioversion
   C. Mediastinal radiation therapy

IV. Diseases of other organs
   A. Pneumonia, pulmonary infarction
   B. Colonic infarction
   C. Metastatic carcinoma of lung or colon

V. Miscellaneous
   A. Sepsis
   B. Shock
   C. Acute psychosis
   D. Hypothyroidism
   E. Bee and wasp stings
   F. Acute asthmatic attack
   G. Macleod syndrome

(From Layzer RB: Diagnosis of neuromuscular disorders. p. 25. In Neuromuscular Manifestations of Systemic Disease. FA Davis, Philadelphia, 1985, with permission.)

Demyelinating Diseases

CLINICAL FEATURES OF MULTIPLE SCLEROSIS

I. Primary (direct effects of demyelination)
- A. Behavioral (euphoria, depression, schizophrenic symptoms)
- B. Weakness
- C. Spasticity
- D. Flexor spasms
- E. Increased deep tendon reflexes
- F. Visual loss
- G. Numbness
- H. Incontinence/sexual dysfunction
- I. Diplopia
- J. Nystagmus (horizontal, upbeating, pendular)
- K. Intranuclear ophthalmoplegia
- L. Oscillopsia
- M. Incoordination
- N. Ataxia
- O. Gait abnormalities
- P. Trigeminal neuralgia
- Q. Facial paralysis
- R. Fatigue
- S. Lhermitte's sign

II. Secondary (to primary signs and symptoms)
- A. Urinary tract infections
- B. Pressure sores
- C. Ankylosis of joints
- D. Fibrous contracture
- E. Aspiration pneumonia

III. Tertiary
- A. Emotional
- B. Social
- C. Vocational
- D. Impact on patient
- E. Impact on family
- F. Impact on community

(From Smith CR, Scheinberg LC: Clinical features of multiple sclerosis. Semin Neurol 5:85–93, 1985, with permission.)

DIAGNOSTIC CRITERIA FOR MULTIPLE SCLEROSIS

I. Clinically definite multiple sclerosis
   A. Two attacks and clinical evidence of two separate lesions
   B. Two attacks; clinical evidence for one lesion and paraclinical (CT, MRI, EP) evidence of another, separate lesion
II. Laboratory-supported definite multiple sclerosis
   The laboratory support is the demonstration in CSF of oligoclonal bands (OB) or increased synthesis of IgG. The serum banding pattern and IgG should be normal. Other causes of CSF changes, such as syphilis, subacute sclerosing panencephalitis, sarcoidosis, collagen vascular disease, and similar disorders, should be excluded.
   A. Two attacks; either clinical or paraclinical evidence of one lesion; and CSF OB/IgG
   B. One attack; clinical evidence of two separate lesions, and CSF OB/IgG
   C. One attack; clinical evidence of one lesion and paraclinical evidence of another, separate lesion; and CSF OB/IgG
III. Clinically probable multiple sclerosis
   A. Two attacks and clinical evidence of one lesion
   B. One attack and clinical evidence of two separate lesions
   C. One attack; clinical evidence of one lesion and paraclinical evidence of another, separate lesion
IV. Laboratory-supported probable multiple sclerosis
   A. Two attacks and CSF OB/IgG

(From Poser CM, Paty DW, Scheinberg L, et al: New diagnostic criteria for multiple sclerosis: guidelines for research protocols. Ann Neurol 13:227–231, 1983, with permission.)

DIFFERENTIAL DIAGNOSIS OF MULTIPLE SCLEROSIS

    I. Acute disseminated encephalomyelitis
    II. Transverse myelitis (may be secondary to viral or bacterial infections)
    III. Leber's optic atrophy
    IV. Hereditary ataxias
    V. Spinocerebellar degeneration
    VI. Tropical spastic paraparesis (HTLV-I infection)
    VII. HIV paraparesis
    VIII. Diffuse sclerosis (Schilder's disease, leukodystrophies)
    IX. Compressive myelopathies
        A. Cervical spondylosis
        B. Spinal cord compression
        C. Platybasia
        D. Basilar impression
        E. Arnold-Chiari malformation
    X. Intracranial tumor—especially brainstem, cerebellum
    XI. Collagen vascular disease (SLE, polyarteritis nodosa)
    XII. CNS vasculitis
    XIII. Neurosyphilis
    XIV. Lyme disease
    XV. Vitamin B_{12} deficiency (gastrectomy, gastric carcinoma, malabsorption syndromes)
    XVI. Motor neuron disease

CLASSIFICATION OF LEUKODYSTROPHIES

    I. Autosomal recessive leukodystrophies
        A. Krabbe's globoid body leukodystrophy
        B. Metachromatic leukodystrophy
    II. X-linked recessive leukodystrophies
        A. Adrenoleukodystrophy
        B. Adrenomyeloneuropathy
        C. Pelizaeus-Merzbacher leukodystrophy
    III. Miscellaneous leukodystrophies
        A. Canavan's disease
        B. Alexander's disease

Neurological Manifestations of Systemic Diseases

NEUROLOGICAL SYNDROMES IN POSTARREST
PATIENTS AWAKENING AFTER PROLONGED COMA

	Cerebral Syndrome	**Spinal Cord Syndrome**
Pathology	Focal or multifocal infarcts especially in boundary zones	Focal or multifocal infarcts of spinal cord
Clinical	Dementia	Flaccid paralysis of lower limbs
	Amnesia	Loss of pain and temperature sense
	Bibrachial paresis	Preserved touch and position sense
	Para- or quadriparesis	Urinary retention
	Visual agnosia	The following may also occur: nonocclusive intestinal ischemia and with bowel infarction
	Cortical blindness The following may also occur: ataxia, seizures, myoclonus, extrapyramidal tract signs	
Outcome	Slow, often incomplete recovery	No or incomplete recovery

(From Caronna JJ: Neurological syndromes following cardiac arrest and cardiac bypass surgery. pp. 707–719. In Barnett HJM et al (eds): Stroke. Churchill Livingstone, New York, 1986, with permission.)

RULES THAT IDENTIFY PATIENTS WITH POOR OR GOOD PROGNOSIS AFTER CARDIAC ARREST

Patients With Virtually No Chance of Regaining Independence:

Time After Cardiac Arrest	Clinical Signs
Initial examination	No pupillary light reflex
1 d	1-d motor response no better than flexor and 1-d spontaneous eye movements are neither orienting nor roving conjugate.
3 d	3-d motor response no better than flexor.
1 wk	1-wk motor response not obeying commands, initial spontaneous eye movements neither orienting nor roving conjugate, and 3-d eye opening not spontaneous.
2 wk	2-wk oculocephalic response not normal, 3-d motor response not obeying commands, 3-d eye opening not spontaneous, and 2-wk eye opening not improved at least two grades.

Patients With Best Chance of Regaining Independence:

Time After Cardiac Arrest	Clinical Signs
Initial examination	Pupillary light reflexes present, motor response and motor response flexor or extensor, and spontaneous eye movements roving conjugate or orienting.
1 d	1-d motor response withdrawal or better and 1-d eye opening improved at least two grades.
3 d	3-d motor response withdrawal or better and 3-d spontaneous eye movements normal.
1 wk	1-wk motor response obeying commands.
2 wk	2-wk oculocephalic response normal.

(From Levy DE, Caronna JJ, Singer BH, et al: Predicting outcome from hypoxic-ischemic coma. JAMA 253:1420–1426, 1985, with permission.)

NEUROLOGICAL SEQUELAE OF CARDIAC SURGERY

I. CNS
   A. Ischemic stroke
   B. Bilateral watershed infarction
   C. Seizures
   D. Subdural hematoma
   E. Epidural hematoma
   F. Intracerebral hematoma
   G. Acute hydrocephalus
   H. Hypoglycemic coma
   I. Acute visual loss
   J. Choreoathetosis
II. Peripheral neuropathy
   A. Saphenous
   B. Peroneal
   C. Phrenic
   D. Ulnar
   E. Recurrent laryngeal
   F. Radial sensory
   G. Facial
   H. Oculosympathetic
   I. Auditory

(From Hotson JR, Enzmann DR: Neurologic complications of cardiac transplantation. Neurol Clin 6:349–365, 1988, with permission.)

HEMATOLOGICAL DISEASES CAUSING NEUROLOGICAL SIGNS OR SYMPTOMS

I. Anemias
   A. Sickle cell anemia
   B. Sickle cell trait
   C. Sickle cell/hemoglobin C disease
   D. Iron deficiency anemia
   E. Hemolytic anemia/extramedullary hematopoiesis
II. Hyperviscosity syndromes
   A. Increased red blood cells
      1. Polycythemia vera
      2. Secondary polycythemia
      3. Benign polycythemia
   B. Increased white blood cells
      1. Hyperleukocytosis
   C. Increased serum proteins (paraproteinemias)
      1. Waldenström's macroglobulinemia
      2. Multiple myeloma
   D. Thrombocytopenia
      1. Immune thrombocytopenia
      2. Thrombotic thrombocytopenia
      3. Heparin-induced
   E. Hemophilia
   F. Disseminated intravascular coagulation
   G. Thrombocythemia
      1. Essential
   H. Hemochromatosis
   I. Anticoagulation
      1. Iatrogenic
      2. Lupus anticoagulants
   J. Vitamin deficiencies
      1. B_1, B_6, B_{12}, A, E

(From Massey EW: Neurological manifestations of hematological disease. Neurol Clin 7:549–561, 1989, with permission.)

NEUROLOGICAL COMPLICATIONS
OF CHEMOTHERAPY

I. Encephalopathy
   A. Methotrexate
   B. Hexamethylmelamine
   C. 5-Fluorouracil
   D. Procarbazine
   E. BCNU
   F. Cisplatin
   G. 5-Azacytidine
   H. Misonidazole
   I. Cytarabine
II. Acute cerebellar syndrome/ataxia
   A. 5-Azacytidine
   B. 5-Fluorouracil
   C. Cytarabine
   D. Procarbazine
   E. Hexamethylmelamine
III. Myelopathy
   A. Intrathecal methotrexate
   B. Intrathecal cytarabine
   C. Intrathecal thiotepa
IV. Neuropathy
   A. Vinca alkaloids
   B. Cisplatin
   C. Hexamethylmelamine
   D. Procarbazine
   E. 5-Azacytidine
   F. Misonidazole
   G. Methyl-G
   H. Cytarabine
V. Cerebral vasculopathy
   A. Cisplatin (arterial)
   B. Asparaginase (venous)

VITAMIN B$_{12}$ DEFICIENCY

   I. Subacute combined degeneration
- A. Posterior columns (sensory disturbances, paresthesias, sensory ataxia, incoordination)
- B. Corticospinal tracts (weakness, spasticity, hyperreflexia)
- C. Spinothalamic tracts (nocturnal cramps, limb pain, abdominal crises, truncal sensory level)

  II. Brain
- A. Dementia, depression, psychiatric disorders
- B. Irritability, apathy, somnolence, confusion

 III. Optic nerves
- A. Decreased visual acuity
- B. Centrocecal scotoma
- C. Impaired color perception

 IV. Other cranial nerves
- A. Disturbances in smell and taste
- B. Tinnitus
- C. Paralysis of upward gaze

  V. Peripheral neuropathy
- A. Stocking-glove sensory loss
- B. Arreflexia

 VI. Autonomic dysfunction
- A. Orthostatic hypotension
- B. Sphincter disturbances
- C. Impotence

VII. Atypical manifestations also described in infants
- A. Mental retardation
- B. Involuntary movements

NEUROLOGICAL SYNDROMES ASSOCIATED WITH HYPERTHYROIDISM

I. Cognitive and behavioral
   A. Nervousness and fatigue
   B. Restlessness and irritability
   C. Manic psychosis
   D. Exacerbation of underlying psychiatric disease
   E. Apathetic thyrotoxicosis (in elderly)
II. Seizures
III. Abnormal movements
   A. Exaggerated essential/physiological tremor
   B. Chorea
IV. Corticospinal tract
   A. Hyperreflexia
   B. Clonus
   C. Spasticity
   D. Babinski response
V. Ophthalmological
   A. Lid lag and upper lid retraction
   B. Proptosis
   C. Extraocular muscle myopathy
   D. Optic nerve compression
VI. Cranial nerve
   A. Bulbar palsy
VII. Neuromuscular
   A. Myopathy
   B. Myokymia
   C. ?Greater incidence of myasthenia gravis
   D. ?Motor polyneuropathy
   E. Thyrotoxic periodic paralysis

(From Kaminski J, Ruff RL: Neurological complications of endocrine diseases. Neurol Clin 7:489–508, 1989, with permission.)

NEUROLOGICAL SYNDROMES ASSOCIATED
WITH HYPOTHYROIDISM

  I. Cognitive and behavioral changes
     A. Fatigue, apathy, inattention
     B. Decreased psychomotor activity
     C. Dementia
     D. Psychosis
     E. Coma
 II. Seizures
     A. Higher frequency of seizures
     B. EEG slowing and decreased amplitude
III. Sleep apnea
     A. Obstructive (secondary to obesity/myxedema)
 IV. Cerebellar
     A. Ataxia and other "cerebellar signs"
     B. Gait ataxia
  V. Cranial nerve
     A. Sensorineural hearing loss
     B. Ptosis
     C. Visual field defects (compression from enlarged pituitary)
 VI. Neuromuscular
     A. Slowed (hung-up) reflexes
     B. Myoedema
     C. Muscle enlargement
     D. Myopathy
     E. Carpal tunnel syndrome
     F. Peripheral neuropathy
     G. Pseudomyotonia
VII. Miscellaneous
     A. Hypothermia
     B. Somnolence

(From Kaminski HJ, Ruff RL: Neurological complications of endocrine diseases. Neurol Clin 7:489–508, 1989, with permission.)

NEUROLOGICAL SYNDROMES ASSOCIATED WITH PARATHYROID ABNORMALITIES

I. Hyperparathyroidism
  A. Cognitive and behavioral
    1. Psychiatric
      a. Mania
      b. Schizophrenia
    2. Acute confusional state
    3. Distractibility
    4. Mental slowness
    5. Neuropsychiatric (dominant hemisphere functions)
  B. Nerve root compression (secondary to vertebral collapse)
  C. Myopathy
    1. Secondary to elevated parathyroid hormone
    2. Impaired activation of vitamin D
II. Hypoparathyroidism
  A. Psychological symptoms
  B. Intellectual impairment
  C. Schizophrenia
  D. Mania
  E. Dementia
  F. Seizures
  G. Basal ganglia calcification
  H. Chorea
  I. Hyperexcitability of nerves
    1. Paresthesias
    2. Carpopedal spasm
    3. Diffuse muscle cramping
    4. Laryngeal spasm
  J. Myopathy

(From Kaminski HJ, Ruff RL: Neurological complications of endocrine diseases. Neurol Clin 7:489–508, 1989, with permission.)

NEUROLOGICAL SYNDROMES ASSOCIATED WITH GLUCOCORTICOID EXCESS

  I. Cognitive and behavioral changes
     A. Psychiatric
        1. Depression
        2. Schizophreniform disorder
        3. Mania
     B. Diffuse cognitive impairment
 II. Spinal cord compression (secondary to excess epidural fat)
III. Cranial nerve
     A. Optic atrophy
     B. Visual field defects
 IV. ?Guillain-Barré syndrome
  V. Myopathy
 VI. Myalgias

(From Kaminski HJ, Ruff RL: Neurological complications of endocrine diseases. Neurol Clin 7:489–508, 1989, with permission.)

NEUROLOGICAL SYNDROMES ASSOCIATED
WITH DIABETES

I. Nonketotic hyperosmolar coma
   A. Focal neurological signs (mimicking stroke)
   B. Motor seizures (including epilepsia partialis continua)
II. Diabetic ketoacidosis
   A. Clouding of consciousness → coma
   B. Generalized weakness
III. Stroke
IV. Neuropathy
   A. Symmetric polyneuropathy
      1. Sensory or sensorimotor polyneuropathy
      2. Acute or subacute motor neuropathy
      3. Autonomic neuropathy
         a. Pupillary and lacrimal dysfunction
         b. Impairment of sweating
         c. Impairment of vascular reflexes
         d. Nocturnal diarrhea
         e. Atonicity of GI tract and bladder
         f. Sexual impotence
         g. Postural hypotension
   B. Focal and multifocal neuropathies
      1. Cranial neuropathy (CN III most common)
      2. Trunk (radiculopathy) and limb neuropathy
      3. Proximal motor neuropathy
V. Retinopathy
VI. Susceptible to CNS infections
   A. Mucormycosis
   B. Aspergillosis
VII. Maternal diabetes
   A. Fetal microcephaly
   B. Fetal myelodysplasia

(From Kaminski HJ, Ruff RL: Neurological complications of endocrine diseases. Neurol Clin 7:489–508, 1989, with permission.)

NEUROLOGICAL MANIFESTATIONS OF RENAL FAILURE

   I. Uremic encephalopathy (confusion, stupor, coma)
  II. Asterixis
 III. Tremor
  IV. Myoclonus
   V. Tetany
  VI. Seizures
 VII. Meningeal signs, CSF pleocytosis
VIII. Neuropathy (distal polyneuropathy, autonomic, cranial)
  IX. Restless-leg syndrome
   X. Dialysis dysequilibrium syndrome
  XI. Dialysis dementia
 XII. Subdural hematoma
XIII. Wernicke's encephalopathy
 XIV. Complications in renal transplant patients
       A. Neoplasm
          1. CNS lymphoma
          2. Metastatic carcinoma
       B. Infection
          1. Fungi
             a. *Cryptococcus*
             b. *Aspergillus*
             c. *Candida*
             d. *Nocardia*
             e. *Histoplasma*
          2. Toxoplasmosis
          3. CMV
       C. Demyelination
          1. Central pontine myelinolysis

(Data from Raskin NH, Fishman RA: Neurological disorders in renal failure. N Engl J Med 294:143–148, 1976, and Fraser, Arieff: Nervous system complications of uremia. Ann Intern Med 109:143–153, 1988.)

NEUROLOGICAL COMPLICATIONS OF RENAL DIALYSIS

   I. Dialysis dementia
  II. Metabolic encephalopathies
     A. Hypercalcemia
     B. Hypophosphatemia
     C. Wernicke's encephalopathy
     D. Hyperosmolarity
     E. Hyponatremia
     F. Drug intoxications
     G. Trace element intoxications: manganese, mercury, lead, nickel, thallium, boron, vanadium, chromium, tin, cadmium
     H. Hyperparathyroidism
 III. Stroke
 IV. Hypertensive encephalopathy
  V. Structural lesions
     A. Subdural hematoma
     B. Normal pressure hydrocephalus
     C. Cerebral hematoma
 VI. Dialysis dysequilibrium syndrome
     A. Acute trace element intoxication (copper, nickel)
     B. Subdural hematoma
     C. Uremia
     D. Nonketotic hyperosmolar coma
     E. Cerebral embolus secondary to shunt declotting
     F. Acute stroke
     G. Cardiac arrhythmia
     H. Depletion syndrome
     I. Malfunction of fluid proportioning system
     J. Excessive ultrafiltration
     K. Hypoglycemia

(Modified from Fraser CL, Arieff AI: Nervous system complications of uremia. Ann Intern Med 109:143–153, 1988, with permission.)

HEPATIC ENCEPHALOPATHY

Stage	Mental Status/Behavior	Motor/Reflexes
1	Mild confusion Anxiety Agitation Diminished attention Impaired serial sevens Altered sleep patterns Depression	Fine postural tremor Slowed coordination
2	Drowsiness Lethargy Gross personality changes Disorientation (time) Poor recall Inappropriate behavior	Asterixis Dysarthria Primitive reflexes (suck, grasp) Paratonia Ataxia
3	Delirium or profound confusion Paranoia Disorientation (time and place) Incomprehensible speech Somnolent, but arousable	Hyperreflexia Seizures Babinski sign Hyperventilation Incontinence Hypothermia Myoclonus
4	Coma	Decerebrate posturing Brisk oculocephalic reflexes

(From Rothstein JD, Herlong HF: Neurological manifestations of hepatic disease. Neurol Clin **7**:563–578, 1989, with permission.)

NEUROLOGICAL COMPLICATIONS
OF ALCOHOL USE

  I. Acute intoxication
   A. Drunkenness (blood concentrations >100 mg/dl [21.7 mmol/L]; nystagmus, diplopia, dysarthria, and ataxia)
   B. Excitement (pathological intoxication)
   C. Blackouts
   D. Coma
 II. Abstinence or withdrawal syndromes
   A. Tremulousness
   B. Hallucinosis
   C. Seizures
   D. Delirium tremens (severe confusional state characterized by agitation, insomnia, hallucinations or dellusions, tremor, and signs of autonomic activity)
III. Nutritional deficiencies
   A. Wernicke's encephalopathy (classic triad: encephalopathy, ophthalmoplegia, and ataxia)
   B. Korsakoff syndrome (marked deficits in memory and apathy with an intact sensorium and normal intellectual functions)
   C. Polyneuropathy
   D. Optic neuropathy ("tobacco-alcohol amblyopia")
   E. Pellagra
 IV. Uncertain pathogenesis, associated with alcohol use
   A. Dementia
   B. Cerebral atrophy
   C. Cerebellar degeneration
   D. Marchiafava-Bignami syndrome
   E. Central pontine myelinolysis
   F. Alcoholic cardiomyopathy
   G. Myopathy
  V. Fetal alcohol syndrome (pre- and postnatal growth retardation, microcephaly, facial dysmorphology, neurological and other congenital anomalies)
 VI. Neurological disorders consequent to Laennec cirrhosis and portal-systemic shunts
   A. Hepatic encephalopathy
   B. Chronic hepatocerebral degeneration

NEUROLOGICAL SYNDROMES ASSOCIATED WITH LUPUS ANTICOAGULANT AND ANTICARDIOLIPIN ANTIBODIES

I. Focal cerebral ischemia
    A. Transient ischemic attack
    B. Ischemic infarction
    C. Cerebral venous thrombosis
II. Dementia
III. Ocular ischemia
    A. Amaurosis fugax
    B. Retinal vein thrombosis
    C. Retinal artery thrombosis
    D. Central retinal artery occlusion
    E. Cilioretinal artery occlusion
    F. Choroidal infarction
IV. Myelopathy
    A. Lupoid sclerosis/Jamaican neuropathy
    B. Kohlmeier-Degos disease
V. Guillain-Barré syndrome
VI. Migraine and migrainous phenomena
    A. Common migraine
    B. Classical migraine
    C. Isolated migrainous scotoma
    D. Fortification spectra
    E. Hemianopic migraine
    F. ?Transient global amnesia
    G. Complicated migraine

NEUROLOGICAL SYNDROMES ASSOCIATED WITH LUPUS ANTICOAGULANT AND ANTICARDIOLIPIN ANTIBODIES (*Continued*)

VII. Chorea
VIII. Seizures
  IX. Inclusion body myositis
   X. ?Neurological manifestations of the following:
    A. Behçet syndrome
    B. Sneddon's disease
    C. Lyme disease
  XI. Systemic manifestations
    A. Coronary thrombosis
    B. Peripheral arterial thrombosis
    C. Recurrent venous thrombosis
    D. Leg ulceration
    E. Livedo reticularis
    F. Spontaneous abortion
    G. Pulmonary hypertension
    H. Thrombocytopenia

(Data from Levine SR, Welch KMA: The spectrum of neurological disease associated with antiphospholipid antibodies. Arch Neurol 44:876–883, 1987, and Coull BM, Bourdette DN, Goodnight SH, et al: Multiple cerebral infarctions and dementia associated with anticardiolipin antibodies. Stroke 18:1107–1112, 1987.)

NEUROLOGICAL COMPLICATIONS
OF SYSTEMIC LUPUS

I. Neurological
   A. Headache
   B. Seizure
   C. Cranial neuropathy
   D. Stroke
   E. Hemiparesis
   F. Movement disorder (chorea, ataxia, hemiballismus)
   G. Transverse myelitis
   H. Optic neuritis
   I. Aseptic meningitis
   J. Pseudotumor cerebri
   K. Neuromuscular junction disorders
   L. Peripheral neuropathy
II. Psychiatric
   A. Cognitive dysfunction
   B. Organic brain syndrome
   C. Schizophreniform psychosis
   D. Affective disorder

REFLEX SYMPATHETIC DYSTROPHY* — PRECIPITATING FACTORS AND ASSOCIATED DISEASES

I. Peripheral
   A. Soft tissue injury
   B. Arthritides
   C. Infection
   D. Fasciitis, tendonitis, bursitis
   E. Venous or arterial thrombosis
   F. Fractures, sprains, dislocations
   G. Operative procedures
   H. Malignancy
   I. Aortic injury
   J. Myelography, spinal anesthesia
   K. Paravertebral alcohol injection
   L. Postherpetic
   M. Brachial plexopathy, scalenus anterior syndrome
   N. Radiculopathy
   O. Immobilization with cast or splint
   P. Vasculitis
   Q. Myocardial infarction
   R. Weber-Christian disease
   S. Polymyalgia rheumatica
   T. Pulmonary fibrosis
II. Central
   A. Brain tumor
   B. Severe head injury
   C. Cerebral infarction
   D. Subarachnoid hemorrhage
   E. Cervical cord injury
   F. Subacute combined degeneration
   G. Syringomyelia
   H. Poliomyelitis
   I. Amyotrophic lateral sclerosis
III. Other
   A. Idiopathic
   B. Prolonged bedrest
   C. Familial

* This syndrome is characterized by burning pain, hyperesthesia, swelling, hyperhidrosis, and trophic changes in the skin and bone of an arm or leg.
(From Schwartzman RJ, McLellan TL: Reflex sympathetic dystrophy. Arch Neurol 44:555–561, 1987, with permission.)

7
NEURO-OPHTHALMOLOGY

CAUSES OF HORNER SYNDROME

I. First-order neuron
   (Hypothalamus to upper thoracic cord)
   A. Brainstem stroke (especially lateral medulla)
   B. Neck trauma
   C. Spinal cord tumor
   D. Syringomyelia
   E. Demyelinating disease

II. Second-order neuron
   (Intermediolateral column in upper cord to superior cervical ganglion)
   A. Neck trauma
   B. Postoperative from neck surgery
   C. Neck mass (abcess, thyroid, lymph nodes)
   D. Vertebral neoplasm
   E. Apical lung lesions (Pancoast's tumor)
   F. Cervical rib
   G. Neurofibroma

III. Third-order neuron
   (Superior cervical ganglion along carotid tree to orbit)
   A. Migraine
   B. Carotid trauma
   C. Carotid dissection
   D. Cavernous sinus lesion
   E. Nasopharyngeal carcinoma
   F. Superior orbital fissure lesion

PUPILLARY SYNDROMES

I. Horner syndrome
   A. Partial ptosis of upper and lower lids
   B. Miosis (usually more marked in dim light)
   C. Variable anhidrosis
   D. Narrowed palpebral fissure, but no true enophthalmos
   E. Transient dilation of facial and conjunctival vessels
   F. Transient ocular hypotony
   G. Transient increased accommodation
   H. Change in tear viscosity
   I. Iris heterochromia (if long-standing)
II. Adie's tonic pupil
   A. Initially unilateral (80%)
   B. Relative mydriasis in bright light
   C. Poor or absent reaction to light
   D. Strong and tonic contraction to near effort
   E. Slow redilation after near effort
   F. Sector palsies of iris
   G. Tonic accommodation
   H. Cholinergic supersensitivity (often associated with diminished deep tendon reflexes)
III. Argyll Robertson pupil
   A. Intact visual function
   B. Decreased pupillary light reaction
   C. Intact near response
   D. Miosis
   E. Irregular pupils
   F. Usually bilateral and unequal
   G. Dilates poorly in dark and in response to mydriatics
   H. Iris atrophy may be present
IV. Hutchinson's pupil
   A. Poorly reactive, dilated pupil of third nerve compression
V. Isolated pupillary dilation
   A. Mydriatic agents
   B. Adie's pupil
   C. Migraine
   D. Contralateral pupillary constriction (e.g., Horner syndrome)
   E. Compression of CN III
      1. Aneurysm
      2. Uncal herniation
   F. Uveitis

OPTIC NEUROPATHY

   I. Vascular (ischemic optic neuropathy)
      A. Arteritic
      B. Nonarteritic
  II. Structural/infiltrative
      A. Optic nerve glioma
      B. Tumor (meningioma, leukemia, lymphoma, sarcoid, metastatic)
      C. Aneurysm
      D. Chronic papilledema
      E. Glaucoma
 III. Myelin
      A. Multiple sclerosis
      B. Postinfectious
  IV. Metabolic
      A. Toxic
      B. Nutritional
   V. Paraneoplastic
  VI. Hereditary/neurodegenerative
      A. Leber's optic neuropathy
      B. Recessive or dominantly inherited optic atrophy
 VII. Inherited neurometabolic disorder
      A. Adrenoleukodystrophy
      B. Krabbe's globoid body leukodystrophy
      C. Metachromatic leukodystrophy
      D. Infantile neuronal ceroid-lipofuscinosis (Santavuori-Haltia)
      E. Friedreich's ataxia
VIII. Trauma

UNILATERAL PROPTOSIS

    I. Thyroid ophthalmopathy
   II. Orbital pseudotumor
  III. Metastasis
  IV. Extension of intracranial neoplasm
   V. Cavernous angioma
  VI. Lymphagioma
 VII. Lacrimal gland tumor
VIII. Lymphoma
  IX. Meningioma
   X. Epidermoid cyst
  XI. Dermoid cyst

CORTICAL VISUAL SYNDROMES

  I. Cortical blindness
    A. With (Anton syndrome) or without denial
 II. Disorders of form analysis
    A. Visual (object) agnosia
    B. Prosopagnosia (inability to visually identify faces)
    C. Alexia without agraphia
    D. Palinopsia (persistence of image once object has been removed)
    E. Illusions/hallucinations
III. Disorders of color analysis
    A. Central achromatopsia
    B. Color anomia
    C. Color memory disturbances
IV. Disorders of spatial analysis
    A. Balint syndrome
      1. Simultanagnosia (inability to recognize the meaning of the whole)
      2. Defects in visually guided limb movements (optic ataxia)
      3. Oculomotor apraxia
    B. Pursuit/OKN defects
    C. Dressing apraxia
    D. Visuospatial disorientation
    E. Visuoconstructive defects
    F. Defective stereopsis

8
PEDIATRIC
NEUROLOGY

COMMON NEWBORN REFLEXES

Reflex	Appears	Disappears	Description
Moro's reflex	Birth	3–5 mo	Abduction of arms, extension of legs, and flexion of hips in response to change in head position
Grasp	Birth	3 mo	Hand or foot grasp to tactile stimuli
Babinski reflex	Birth	8–18 mo	Great toe extension (flexion of other toes) with stimulation of sole of foot
Stepping reflex	Birth	1–2 mo	Dorsal surface of the foot is brushed on the underside of a tabletop; the baby flexes the hip and knee (as if attempting to step onto the table)
Tonic neck reflexes	Birth	3 mo	Turning head to side leads to extension of ipsilateral arm and leg, with contralateral flexion— should be transient
Sucking	Birth	4 mo	Baby sucks on objects placed in mouth
Landau reflex	3 mo	18 mo	The infant is held in the prone position and extends the neck, trunk, and legs
Neck righting	5 mo	2 yr	When the baby's head is turned to one side, the trunk is rolled to the same side

NEONATAL SEIZURES—DIFFERENTIAL DIAGNOSIS
BY PEAK TIME OF ONSET

I. 24 hours
   - A. Bacterial meningitis, sepsis
   - B. Drugs
   - C. Hypoxic/ischemic encephalopathy
   - D. Intrauterine infection
   - E. Intraventricular hemorrhage at term
   - F. Laceration of tentorium or falx
   - G. Pyridoxine dependency
   - H. Subarachnoid hemorrhage

II. 24 to 72 hours
   - A. Bacterial meningitis, sepsis
   - B. Cerebral contusion with subdural hemorrhage
   - C. Cerebral dysgenesis
   - D. Cerebral infarction
   - E. Drug withdrawal
   - F. Glycine encephalopathy
   - G. Glycogen synthase deficiency
   - H. Hypoparathyroidism-hypocalcemia
   - I. Hypoglycemia
   - J. Incontinentia pigmenti
   - K. Intracerebral hemorrhage
   - L. Intraventricular hemorrhagee in premature infants
   - M. Pyridoxine dependency
   - N. Subarachnoid hemorrhage
   - O. Tuberous sclerosis
   - P. Urea cycle disorders

III. 72 hours to 1 week
   - A. Benign familial neonatal convulsions
   - B. Cerebral dysgenesis
   - C. Cerebral infarction
   - D. Hypoparathyroidism
   - E. Intracerebral hemorrhage
   - F. Kernicterus
   - G. Ketotic hyperglycinemias
   - H. Nutritional hypocalcemia
   - I. Tuberous sclerosis
   - J. Urea cycle disorders

IV. 1 to 4 weeks
   - A. Adrenoleukodystrophy, neonatal form
   - B. Cerebral dysgenesis

NEONATAL SEIZURES—DIFFERENTIAL DIAGNOSIS
BY PEAK TIME OF ONSET (*Continued*)

  C. Fructose dysmetabolism
  D. Gaucher's disease
  E. Infantile GM_1 gangliosidosis
  F. Herpes simplex encephalitis
  G. Ketotic hyperglycinemias
  H. Maple syrup urine disease
  I. Mitochondrial disorders
  J. Tuberous sclerosis
  K. Urea cycle disorders

(From Fenichel GM: Seizures. p. 17. In Clinical Pediatric Neurology. WB Saunders, Philadelphia, 1988, with permission.)

LABORATORY SCREENING TESTS FOR INHERITED NEUROMETABOLIC DISORDERS CAUSING NEONATAL SEIZURES

I. Blood glucose low
   A. Fructose-1,6-diphosphatase deficiency
   B. Glycogen storage disease, type I
   C. Maple syrup urine disease
II. Serum calcium low
   A. Hypoparathyroidism
   B. Maternal hyperparathyroidism
III. Serum ammonia high
   A. Argininosuccinic acidemia
   B. Carbamyl phosphate synthetase deficiency
   C. Citrullinemia
   D. Ornithine transcarbamylase deficiency
   E. Methylmalonic acidemia (may be normal)
   F. Multiple carboxylase deficiency
   G. Propionic acidemia (may be normal)
IV. Serum lactate high
   A. Fructose-1,6-diphosphatase deficiency
   B. Glycogen storage disease, type I
   C. Multiple carboxylase deficiency
   D. Pyruvate carboxylase deficiency
   E. Pyruvate dehydrogenase complex disorders
V. Metabolic acidosis
   A. Fructose-1,6-diphosphatase deficiency
   B. Glycogen storage disease, type I
   C. Maple syrup urine disease
   D. Methylmalonic acidemia
   E. Multiple carboxylase deficiency
   F. Propionic acidemia
   G. Pyruvate carboxylase deficiency
   H. Pyruvate dehydrogenase complex disorders
VI. Urine ferric chloride or dinitrophenylhydrazine
   A. Maple syrup urine disease
VII. No rapid screening test
   A. Adrenoleukodystrophy, neonatal form
   B. Glycine encephalopathy
   C. Glycogen synthase deficiency
   D. Infantile GM_1 gangliosidosis

(From Fenichel GM: Seizures. p. 17. In Clinical Pediatric Neurology. WB Saunders, Philadelphia, 1988, with permission.)

ANTICONVULSANT THERAPY IN CHILDREN*

Drug	Dose (mg/kg/d)	Schedule (doses/day)	Thera-peutic Blood level (μmol/L)	Seizure Type[†]	Complications
Diphenylhydantoin (Dilantin)	5–10	1–2	10–20 (37–73)	GM, PAR, MM	Gingival hypertrophy, hirsutism, rash, mononucleosis-like reaction, bone marrow suppression, megaloblastic anemia
Phenobarbital	3–5	1–2	15–30 (65–130)	GM, PAR, MM	Hyperactivity, impaired learning, depression
Primidone (Mysoline)	10–20	2–3	5–15 (23–69)	GM, PAR	Same as for phenobarbital
Carbamazepine (Tegretol)	20–30	2–3	6–12 (25–50)	GM, PAR, MM	Bone marrow suppression, neutropenia, hepatic injury

* The drugs listed are the most commonly used anticonvulsants.
† GM, generalized motor; PAR, partial; MM, minor motor; PM, petit mal.
(Modified from Evans OB: Seizures and epilepsy. p. 387. In Manual of Child Neurology. Churchill Livingstone, New York, 1987, with permission.)

List Continues

335

ANTICONVULSANT THERAPY IN CHILDREN* (*Continued*)

Drug	Dose (mg/kg/d)	Schedule (doses/day)	Therapeutic Blood level (μmol/L)	Seizure Type[†]	Complications
Valproic acid (Depakene)	30–60	3–4	50–90 (350–630)	GM, PAR, PM, MM	Hepatic failure (idiosyncratic), hepatic injury (dose related) alopecia, hyperammonemia, tremor, bone marrow suppression, nausea/vomiting, pancreatitis
Valproic acid (Depakote)	20–50	2–3	50–90 (350–630)	GM, PAR, PM, MM	Same as above
Ethosuximide (Zarontin)	20–30	1–2	40–60 (280–425)	PM	Abdominal pain, vomiting, bone marrow suppression, nightmares
Clonazepam (Klonopin)	0.2–0.3	3–4	0.02–0.06 (0.063–0.19)	GM, MM	Depression, altered behavior, drooling

TOPOGRAPHIC DIFFERENTIAL DIAGNOSIS OF INTRACRANIAL TUMORS IN CHILDHOOD— SUPRATENTORIAL

  I. Cerebral hemisphere
     A. Astrocytoma
     B. Ependymoma
     C. Primitive neuroectodermal tumor
     D. Cavernous angioma
     E. Oligodendroglioma
 II. Corpus callosum
     A. Astrocytoma-anaplastic astrocytoma
     B. Lipoma
III. Lateral ventricle
     A. Ependymoma
     B. Choroid plexus papilloma
 IV. Region of the third ventricle
     A. Pilocytic astrocytoma
     B. Ependymoma
     C. Choroid plexus papilloma
  V. Optic chiasm and nerve
     A. Astrocytoma
 VI. Pituitary region
     A. Craniopharyngioma
     B. Germ cell neoplasm
     C. Pituitary adenoma
VII. Pineal region
     A. Germ cell neoplasm
     B. Teratoma
     C. Pineocytoma/pineoblastoma

(From Polachini I: Brain tumors: MR imaging. pp. 39–50. In: American Academy of Neurology, Annual Course #242 (Clinical Neuroimaging), 1990, with permission.)

TOPOGRAPHICAL DIFFERENTIAL DIAGNOSIS OF INTRACRANIAL TUMORS IN CHILDHOOD— INFRATENTORIAL

I. Cerebellum
   A. Medulloblastoma
   B. Astrocytoma
   C. Dermoid cyst
II. Fourth ventricle
   A. Ependymoma
   B. Choroid plexus papilloma
III. Cerebellopontine angle
   A. Ependymoma
   B. Choroid plexus papilloma
IV. Brainstem
   A. Astrocytoma-anaplastic astrocytoma
   B. Venous angioma

(From Polachini I: Brain tumors: MR imaging. pp. 39–50. In: American Academy of Neurology, Annual Course #242 (Clinical Neuroimaging), 1990, with permission.)

MEGALOCEPHALY

I. Hydrocephalus
  A. Noncommunicating
    1. Arnold-Chiari malformation
    2. Aqueductal stenosis
    3. Dandy-Walker syndrome
    4. Neoplasm
    5. Aneurysm of vein of Galen
  B. Communicating
    1. Meningeal fibrosis
      a. Postinflammatory
      b. Posthemorrhagic
    2. Vascular
      a. Ateriovenous fistula
      b. Venous occlusion
    3. Choroid plexus papilloma
    4. Neurocutaneous syndrome
      a. Basal cell carcinoma
      b. Incontinentia pigmenti
    5. Malformation-destructive lesions
      a. Hydranencephaly
      b. Porencephaly
      c. Holoprosencephaly
II. Brain edema (toxic-metabolic)
  A. Intoxication (lead, vitamin A, tetracycline)
  B. Endocrine
    1. Hypoparathyroidism
    2. Hypoadrenocorticism
  C. Galactosemia
  D. Idiopathic—pseudotumor cerebri
III. Subdural fluid
  A. Hematoma
  B. Hygroma
  C. Empyema
IV. Thickened skull
  A. Chronic anemia
  B. Cranioskeletal dysplasia
    1. Rickets
    2. Osteopetrosis
    3. Osteogenesis imperfecta
    4. Hyperphosphatasemia
    5. Epiphyseal dysplasia

List Continues

MEGALOCEPHALY *(Continued)*

V. Megalencephaly (big brain)
  A. Anatomic
    1. Gigantism (Cerebral, pituitary, arachnodactyly, adiposogigantism)
    2. Dwarfism (multiple endocrinopathy, achondroplasia)
    3. Neurocutaneous syndrome (neurofibromatosis, tuberous sclerosis, multiple hemangiomatosis)
    4. Familial megalencephaly (dominant and recessive forms)
  B. Metabolic
    1. Aminoaciduria (maple syrup urine disease)
    2. Leukodystrophy (Canavan's spongy degeneration, Alexander's disease)
    3. Lysosomal diseases (Tay-Sachs disease, generalized gangliosidosis, mucopolysaccharidosis, metachromatic leukodystrophy)
    4. Hypoparathyroidism-hypoadrenocorticism

(From DeMeyer W: Megalencephaly in children. Neurology. 22:634–643, 1972, with permission.)

MICROCEPHALY

I. Genetic
   A. Familial microcephaly (autosomal dominant, autosomal recessive, and X-linked forms)
   B. Hereditary syndromes (nonchromosomal)
      1. Prader-Willi syndrome
      2. Rubinstein-Taybi syndrome
      3. Smith-Lemli-Opitz syndrome
      4. de Lange syndrome
      5. Hallermann-Streiff-François syndrome
      6. Alpers syndrome
      7. Fanconi syndrome
      8. Seckel syndrome
II. Infections
   A. Neonatal meningitis
   B. Encephalitis
III. Metabolic abnormalities
   A. Phenylketonuria
   B. Neonatal hypoglycemia
   C. Maple syrup urine disease
   D. Krabbe's disease
   E. Infantile ceroid-lipofuscinosis
   F. Incontinentia pigmenti
IV. Chromosomal abnormalities
   A. Trisomies 13, 18, 21
V. Deletion syndromes
   A. Cri du chat syndrome
VII. Neurological injury
   A. Hypoxic-ischemic injuries
   B. Intracranial hemorrhage
   C. Malnutrition
VII. Intrauterine injuries
   A. Radiation exposure
   B. Infections
      1. Toxoplasmosis
      2. Rubella
      3. Cytomegalovirus
      4. Herpes simplex
      5. Coxsackie virus (group B)
   C. Diabetes
   D. Uremia

List Continues

MICROCEPHALY (*Continued*)

    E. Malnutrition
    F. Hypertension
    G. Maternal alcohol use
    H. Carbon monoxide
    I. Phenytoin
VIII. Miscellaneous
    A. Rett syndrome
    B. Chronic cardiopulmonary disease
    C. Chronic renal disease
    D. Xeroderma pigmentosum
    E. Craniosynostosis

NEONATAL HYDROCEPHALUS: CAUSES, ASSOCIATIONS, AND CHARACTERISTICS

Cause or Association	Characteristics
Meningomyelocele	Arnold-Chiari deformity, hydrocephalus in 75%
Tumors	Obstruction of flow of CSF pathway by teratoma or increased production by choroid plexus papilloma
X-linked recessive	Aqueductal stenosis
Dominant inheritance	Achondroplasia, osteogenesis imperfecta, tuberous sclerosis, neurofibromatosis
Cerebellar anomalies	Dandy-Walker syndrome
Chromosomal anomalies	Occasionally in trisomy 13 and 18
Prenatal infections	Occasionally in CMV and toxoplasmosis
Cysts	Retrocerebellar arachnoid and neuroepithelial, colloid
Meningeal factors	Melanosis
Vascular anomalies	Aneurysm of vein of Galen

(From Lemire RJ: Neural tube defects. JAMA 259:558–562, 1988, with permission.)

CRANIOSYNOSTOSIS

Primary Head Shape/Syndrome	Suture(s) Affected
Scaphocephaly	Sagittal
Brachycephaly	Coronal
Plagiocephaly	Coronal or lambdoidal or both—unilateral
Trigonocephaly	Metopic
Oxycephaly	Multiple sutures
Alper's syndrome	Coronal and basal skull
Carpenter syndrome	Coronal and basal skull
Crouzon syndrome	Coronal and basal skull

(From Jacobson RI: Abnormalities of the skull in children. Neurol Clin 3:117–145, 1985, with permission.)

CLASSIFICATION OF NEURAL TUBE DEFECTS

Location	Classification	Mechanism	Gestational Age (d)
Prior to neural tube closure			
Craniospinal	Craniorachischisis	Nonfusion of neural folds	17–23
Cranial	Anencephaly	Nonclosure of rostral neuropore or neural folds	23–26
Spinal	Meningomyelocele	Nonclosure of caudal neuropore or neural folds	26–30
After neural tube closure			
Craniospinal	Iniencephaly	Unknown, possibly focal somite damage	30–57
Cranial	Encephalocele	Focal mesodermal defect	26–57
Cranial	Hydrocephalus	Numerous mechanisms	26–birth
Spinal	Lumbosacral	Aberrations of canalization and retrogressive differentiation	30–birth

COMMON NONNEURAL TUBE CNS MALFORMATIONS

Location	Malformation	Mechanism(s)
Cranial	Hydranencephaly	Infections, drugs, vascular, trauma
	Holoprosencephaly	Trisomy 13, 18p-, 13q-, autosomal recessive or dominant; rarely environmental cause
	Microcephaly	Autosomal recessive, many chromosomal anomalies; infection, radiation, alcohol
	Porencephaly	Arrest in development, vascular, infections, perinatal asphyxia
	Agyria	Genetic association, dominant and recessive; arrest of cellular migration
	Agenesis of corpus callosum	Autosomal dominant association, recessive inheritance including X-linked chromosome anomalies
	Cerebellar hypoplasia (Dandy-Walker syndrome)	Arrest in development, occlusions of outlet foramina
	Macroencephaly	Genetic association, found in many syndromes
Spinal	Diastematomyelia	Dural sheaths and bony septum
	Hydromyelia-syringomyelia	Focal arrest in development and degeneration

(From Lemire RJ: Neural tube defects. JAMA 259:558–562, 1988, with permission.)

CLINICAL INDICATIONS FOR CHROMOSOME ANALYSIS

I. Head and neck
   A. Occipital scalp defect
   B. Small or low-set ears
   C. Mongoloid-slant (non-Oriental)
   D. Microphthalmia
   E. Hypertelorism or hypotelorism
   F. High nasal bridge
   G. Small or fish mouth
   H. Small mandible
   I. Webbed neck
II. Limbs
   A. Low-set thumb
   B. Overlapping fingers
   C. Abnormal dermatoglyphics
   D. Rocker-bottom feet
   E. Polydactyly
III. Genitourinary
   A. Polycystic kidney
   B. Ambiguous genitalia

(From Fenichel GM: Psychomotor retardation and regression. p. 121. In Clinical Pediatric Neurology. WB Saunders, Philadelphia, 1988, with permission.)

DIFFERENTIAL DIAGNOSIS OF CEREBRAL PALSY

I. Neuromuscular
  A. Congenital
    1. Myopathies
    2. Myasthenia gravis
    3. Hypomyelinating neuropathies
    4. Spinal muscular atrophy
  B. Postnatal
    1. Muscular dystrophies
    2. Familial polyneuropathies
    3. Myasthenia gravis
    4. Spinal muscular atrophy
II. Degenerative
  A. Familial spastic paraparesis
  B. Friedreich's ataxia and other spinocerebellar degenerations
  C. Childhood Huntington's disease
III. Metabolic
  A. Lysosomal storage disease
  B. Aminoacidurias
  C. Pyruvate dysmetabolism
  D. Metabolic myopathies
  E. Wilson's disease
  F. Many others
IV. Bone and joint deformities
  A. Arthrogryposis mutiplex congenita
  B. Equinovarus deformities
V. Disorders of involuntary movement
  A. Tics/Tourette syndrome
  B. Dystonia musculorum deformans
  C. Torsion dystonia
  E. Sydenham's chorea
  E. Spasmus nutans
  F. Continuous motor activity (Isaacs, stiff-man syndrome)
VI. Myelopathies
  A. Spinal dysraphia
  B. Diastematomyelia
  C. Tethered cord syndrome
  E. Spinal cord tumor, arteriovenous malformation
  E. Malformation of the brain

(From Evans OB: Cerebral palsy. p. 159. In Manual of Child Neurology. Churchill Livingstone, New York, 1987, with permission.)

NEUROCUTANEOUS SYNDROMES

I. Tuberous sclerosis
   A. Seizures (infantile spasms, Lennox-Gastaut syndrome, neonatal seizures, tonic-clonic, simple or complex partial)
   B. Abnormal hair pigmentation
   C. Adenoma sebaceum
   D. Ash-leaf spots
   E. Shagreen patches
   F. Café au lait spots
   G. Autosomal dominant
II. Neurofibromatosis
   A. Seizures (generalized, simple or complex partial)
   B. Café au lait spots
   C. Axillary freckles
   D. Neural tumors (acoustic, trigeminal, spinal root cutaneous nerve neuromas, optic glioma)
   E. Lisch nodule (white iris hamartoma)
   F. Autosomal dominant
III. Sturge-Weber syndrome
   A. Seizures (status, epilepsia partialis continua, simple motor)
   B. Hemifacial hemangioma
   C. Tram-line calcification of parieto-occipital cortex
IV. von Hippel-Lindau syndrome
   A. Retinal angiomatosis
   B. Spinal and cerebellar hemangioblastoma
   C. Polycystic kidneys
   D. Autosomal dominant
V. Osler-Weber-Rendu disease
   A. Multiple telangiectasia and vascular malformations of:
      1. Skin
      2. Mucous membranes
      3. Lungs
      4. Brain
      5. GI tract
      6. Autosomal dominant
VI. Ataxia-telangiectasia
   A. Oculocutaneous telangiectasia
   B. Ataxia
   C. Chorea
   D. Immunodeficiency
   E. Frequent sinopulmonary infections
   F. Autosomal recessive

List Continues

NEUROCUTANEOUS SYNDROMES (*Continued*)

VII. Incontinentia pigmenti
    A. Seizures (neonatal, generalized tonic-clonic)
    B. Erythematous bullae (neonate)
    C. Pigmentary whorls (infant)
    D. Depigmented areas (childhood)
VIII. Albright syndrome
    A. Café au lait spots
    B. Mental retardation
    C. Sporadic inheritance
IX. Klippel-Trenaunay syndrome
    A. Port wine stain
    B. Mental retardation
    C. Limb hypertrophy
    D. Sporadic inheritance
X. Hypomelanosis of Ito
    A. Patterns of hypopigmentation
    B. Seizures
    C. Mental retardation
    D. Sporadic inheritance
XI. Linear nevus sebaceous syndrome
    A. Seizures (infantile spasms, Lennox-Gastaut syndrome, generalized tonic-clonic)
    B. Linear facial sebaceous nevus

ROUTINE ABNORMALITIES ASSOCIATED WITH METABOLIC DISEASES

I. Acidosis, increased anion gap
   A. Organic acidemias
   B. Maple syrup urine disease
   C. Hereditary tyrosinemia
   D. Hereditary fructose intolerance
   E. Fructosuria
   F. Galactosemia

II. Lactic acidosis
   A. Pyruvate dehydrogenase deficiency
   B. Pyruvate carboxylase deficiency
   C. Organic acidurias
   D. Multiple carboxylase deficiency
   E. Mitochondrial encephalomyopathies
   F. Glycogen storage disease type I
   G. Leigh's disease

III. Renal tubular acidosis
   A. Fanconi syndrome
   B. Hereditary tyrosinemia
   C. Galactosemia
   D. Hereditary fructose intolerance
   E. Lowe syndrome
   F. Wilson's disease
   G. Primary renal tubular acidosis

IV. Hypoglycemia
   A. Fructosuria
   B. Hereditary fructose intolerance
   C. Galactosemia
   D. Glucose-6-phosphatase deficiency
   E. Maple syrup urine disease
   F. Hereditary tyrosinemia
   G. Organic acidemias

V. Hyperammonemia
   A. Urea cycle disorders
   B. Organic acidemias

VI. Mellituria (sugar in urine)
   A. Hereditary fructose intolerance
   B. Fructosuria
   C. Galactosemia
   D. Fanconi syndrome

List Continues

ROUTINE ABNORMALITIES ASSOCIATED
WITH METABOLIC DISEASES (*Continued*)

VII. Low blood urea nitrogen
  A. Urea cycle disorders
  B. Hyperuricemia
  C. Lesch-Nyhan syndrome
  D. Hereditary fructose intolerance
  E. Glycogen storage disease type I
VIII. Hyperbilirubinemia
  A. Galactosemia
  B. Hereditary tyrosinemia
  C. Hereditary fructose intolerance
  IX. Elevated AST, ALT
  A. Hereditary tyrosinemia
  B. Wilson's disease
  C. Galactosemia
  D. Hereditary fructose intolerance
  X. Uremia
  A. Fabry's disease
  B. Mucolipidosis
  C. Lesch-Nyhan syndrome
  XI. Anemia, thrombocytopenia
  A. Organic acidurias

(From Evans OB: Overview of metabolic and degenerative diseases. p. 189. Manual of Child Neurology. Churchill Livingstone, New York, 1987, with permission.)

NEONATAL HYPERAMMONEMIA

I. Liver failure
II. Urea cycle defects
    A. Argininosuccinic acidemia
    B. Carbamyl phosphate synthetase deficiency
    C. Citrullinemia
    D. Ornithine transcarbamylase deficiency
III. Amino acid metabolism disorders
    A. Glycine encephalopathy
    B. Isovaleric acidemia
    C. Methylmalonic acidemia
    D. Multiple carboxylase deficiency
    E. Propionic acidemia
IV. Transient hyperammonemia of prematurity

(From Fenichel GM: Paroxysmal disorders. p. 13. In Clinical Pediatric Neurology. WB Saunders, Philadelphia, 1988, with permission.)

DIAGNOSTIC CRITERIA FOR REYE SYNDROME

I. Presence of an antecedent viral infection
II. Latent interval of several days before onset of pernicious vomiting
III. Development of a diffuse encephalopathy
IV. No other explanation for encephalopathy
V. Threefold or greater elevation of serum transaminase activities
VI. Prolongation of prothrombin time
VII. Hyperammonemia
VIII. Normal CSF examination

(From Fishman MA: p. 355. Pediatric Neurology. Orlando, Grune & Stratton, FL, 1986, with permission.)

REYE-LIKE SYNDROMES

 I. Urea cycle disorders
  A. Arginase deficiency
  B. *N*-acetylglutamate synthetase deficiency
  C. Argininosuccinic acidemia
  D. Carbamyl phosphate synthetase deficiency
  E. Ornithine transcarbamylase deficiency
 II. Triple-H syndrome
  A. Hyperammonemia
  B. Hyperornithinemia
  C. Homocitrullinuria
 III. Organic aciduria
 IV. Amino acid metabolism disorders
  A. Isovaleric acidemia
  B. Glutaric aciduria
 V. Fatty acid oxidation disorders
  A. Acyl coenzyme A dehydrogenase deficiencies
 VI. Systemic carnitine deficiency
 VII. Fructosemia

(Modified from Crichley EMR: Neurological Emergencies. WB Saunders, London, 1988, with permission.)

INFANTILE HYPOTONIA

I. Cerebral hypotonia
  A. Acute perinatal encephalopathy
    1. Perinatal asphyxia
    2. Sepsis and meningitis
    3. Acquired metabolic disturbances of glucose, calcium, and electrolytes
    4. Inborn errors of metabolism
    5. Birth trauma
    6. Intracranial hemorrhage
    7. Intoxication
    8. Drug withdrawal
  B. Chronic encephalopathy
    1. Neural tube defects
    2. Microcephaly
    3. Cerebral and cerebellar malformations
    4. Chromosomal disorders
    5. Congenital infections
    6. Dysmorphic syndromes
      a. Prader-Willi syndrome
      b. Cohen syndrome
      c. Zellweger syndrome
      d. Lowe syndrome
II. Myelopathy
  A. Trauma
  B. Malformations
III. Spinal muscular atrophy
  A. Werdnig-Hoffman disease
  B. Neurogenic arthrogryposis
IV. Polyneuropathy
  A. Congenital hypomyelinating polyneuropathy
  B. Hereditary sensory neuropathy
  C. Familial dysautonomia (Riley-Day syndrome)
V. Myasthenic disorders
  A. Transitory neonatal myasthenia gravis
  B. Congenital myasthenias
  C. Infantile botulism

List Continues

INFANTILE HYPOTONIA (*Continued*)

VI. Myopathies
  A. Myotonic dystrophy
  B. Congenital muscular dystrophy
  C. Congenital myopathies with fiber type disproportion
  D. Metabolic myopathies

(From Evans OB: The floppy infant. p. 111. In Manual of Child Neurology. Churchill Livingstone, New York, 1987, with permission.)

EYE ABNORMALITIES IN NEUROLOGIC DISEASE

Examination	Sign	Neurological Disorder
Optic disc	Papilledema	Increased intracranial pressure (any cause)
		Acute optic neuritis (papillitis)
		Pseudopapilledema (often hereditary)
		Retro-orbital mass
	Optic atrophy	Demyelinating diseases (many)
		Chronic papilledema
		Leber's optic atrophy
		Neuronal ceroid lipofuscinosis
		Congenital infections (vasculitis, glaucoma)
		Leukodystrophies
Retina	Pigmentation	Congenital infection
		Refsum's disease
		Abetalipoproteinemia
		Neuronal ceroid lipofuscinosis
		Sjögren-Larsson syndrome
		Cockayne syndrome
		Laurence-Moon-Biedl syndrome
		Chédiak-Higashi syndrome
	Colobomas	Aicardi syndrome
	Hemangiomas	von Hippel-Lindau syndrome
	Cherry-red spot	Tay-Sachs disease
		Gangliosidoses
		Sialidoses, mucolipidoses
		Niemann-Pick disease
		Cherry-red spot, myoclonus syndrome
		Metachromatic leukodystrophy
		Farber's lipogranulomatosis
		Central retinal artery occlusion
		Trauma
	Phakomas	Tuberous sclerosis

List Continues

EYE ABNORMALITIES IN NEUROLOGIC DISEASE
(*Continued*)

Exami-nation	Sign	Neurological Disorder
Lens	Cataracts	Conradi syndrome
		Cockayne syndrome
		Lowe syndrome
		Marinesco-Sjögren syndrome
		Hallermann-Streiff syndrome
		Pierre Robin syndrome
		Treacher Collins syndrome
		Goldenhar syndrome
		Alport syndrome
		Cerebrotendinous xanthomatosis
		Trisomy 13,18,21
		Incontinentia pigmenti
		Congenital infections
		Familial
		Galactosemia
		Myotonic dystrophy
		Congenital hypothyroidism
		Idiopathic
	Subluxation	Homocystinuria
		Marfan syndrome
		Sulfite oxidase deficiency
Cornea	Clouding	Mucopolysaccharidoses
		Fabry syndrome
		Congenital rubella
Sclera	Telangiectasia	Ataxia telangiectasia
Iris	Pigmentation	Kayser-Fleischer rings (Wilson's disease)
		Brushfield spots (Down syndrome)
	Aniridia	Cerebellar aplasia (Gillespie syndrome)

(From Evans OB: General physical examination. p. 19. In Manual of Child Neurology. Churchill Livingstone, New York, 1987, with permission.)

9
NEURO-
DIAGNOSTIC
PROCEDURES

TESTS ON CSF

I. Routine
   A. Cell count (total and differential)
   B. Glucose level determination
   C. Protein level determination
II. When indicated
   A. Cell count on more than one tube
   B. VDRL for syphilis
   C. Lyme titers
   D. Protein electrophoresis
   E. Assay for fungal antigens
   F. Cultures
      1. Bacteria
      2. Fungi
      3. Viruses
      4. *Mycobacterium tuberculosis*
   G. Stains
      1. Gram stain for bacteria
      2. Smear for acid-fast organisms
      3. Cytologic examination
   H. Specialized (limited availability)
      1. Spectrophotometry
      2. Assay for bacterial antigens
      3. Assay for myelin basic protein

(From Marton KI, Gean AD: The spinal tap: a new look at an old test. Ann Intern Med 104:840–848, 1986, with permission.)

DISEASES ASSOCIATED WITH
HYPOGLYCORRHACHIA (LOW CSF GLUCOSE)

I. Bacterial meningitis
   A. Pyogenic meningitis
   B. Tuberculosis
   C. Syphilis
   D. Leptospirosis
   E. Brucellosis
II. Neoplasia
III. Subarachnoid hemorrhage
IV. Sarcoidosis
V. Fungal infections
   A. Cryptococcus
   B. Histoplasmosis
   C. Blastomycosis
VI. Viral meningoencephalitis
   A. Lymphocytic choriomeningitis
   B. Mumps
   C. Herpes simplex
VII. Mollaret's meningitis
VIII. Benign lymphocytic meningitis
IX. Epidermoid cyst
X. Intracranial infections
   A. Brain abscess
   B. Septic emboli (endocarditis)
XI. Diabetic ketoacidosis
XII. Systemic hypoglycemia
XIII. Reye syndrome

(From Ellner JJ, Bennett JE: Chronic meningitis. Medicine 55:341–369, 1976, with permission.)

INCREASED CSF PROTEIN

    I. Bacterial meningitis
   II. Viral encephalitis
  III. Syphilis
  IV. Neoplasia (primary, metastatic)
   V. Abscess
  VI. Subdural hematoma
 VII. Polyneuropathy (diphtheria)
VIII. Myxedema
  IX. Diabetes mellitus
   X. Hyperparathyroidism
  XI. Fungal meningitis*
 XII. Tuberculous meningitis*
XIII. Spinal-subarachnoid block*
XIV. Guillian-Barré syndrome*

* May be associated with very high protein.

CSF OLIGOCLONAL BANDS*

    I. Multiple sclerosis
  II. Subacute sclerosing panencephalitis
 III. Guillian-Barré syndrome
 IV. Neurosyphilis
   V. Infections (especially herpes simplex encephalitis)
 VI. Infrequently seen with the following:
    A. Peripheral neuropathy (5% of cases)
    B. CNS tumors (4% of cases)
    C. Stroke (2% of cases)
    D. Alzheimer's disease
    E. Idiopathic vertigo
    F. Epilepsy
    G. Amyotrophic lateral sclerosis

* Oligoclonal bands are seen after electrophoresis of CSF and staining of IgG region. A pattern of banding may be seen even when the total CSF IgG content is normal.

NORMAL EEG PATTERNS

I. Frequency categories
   A. Alpha: 8–13 Hz
   B. Beta: >13 Hz
   C. Theta: 4–7 Hz
   D. Delta: <4 Hz
II. Stages of sleep
   A. Drowsiness
      1. Increase in background slowing
      2. Positive occipital sharp transients of sleep (POSTS)
      3. Small sharp spikes
   B. Stage I sleep
      1. Increase in background slowing
      2. Attenuation of alpha activity
      3. V waves
   C. Stage II sleep
      1. V waves
      2. K complexes
      3. Sleep spindles
   D. Stage III sleep
      1. Increase in delta activity (<50%)
      2. Progressively less sleep spindles
   E. Stage IV sleep
      1. Increase in delta activity (>50%)
      2. Few sleep spindles
   F. REM sleep
      1. Low amplitude mixed frequency (theta and alpha)
      2. Eye movements
      3. Irregular respiration
III. Normal variants
   A. Slow alpha variant
      1. Usually half the normal alpha frequency
   B. Benign epileptiform transients of sleep (small sharp spikes)
      1. Diphasic spike
      2. Little or no following slow wave

NORMAL EEG PATTERNS (*Continued*)

C. Psychomotor variant (rhythmic midtemporal theta)
1. Notched rhythmic theta over temporal regions in drowsiness
D. 6/s spike and wave
1. Small spikes, large slow waves occur in generalized bursts of <1 second
E. Fourteen and six positive spikes
1. Rhythmic bursts of surface positive sharp waves
2. Associated with 6/s spike and wave
F. Wickets
1. Temporal mu rhythm seen in drowsiness
G. Subclinical rhythmic epileptiform discharges of adults (SREDA)
1. Rare variant
2. Runs of sharp theta over central and parietal regions
3. May last minutes
4. No correlation with epilepsy

IV. Activation procedures
A. Hyperventilation
1. Produces symmetrical slowing
2. May activate epileptiform foci or accentuate focal slowing secondary to a structural lesion
3. Contraindicated in recent MI, stroke, sickle cell disease
B. Photic stimulation
1. Evoked occipital activity, usually asymmetrical
2. Photoconvulsive response
a. Paroxysmal burst of spike and wave, not necessarily time locked to stimulus frequency
b. Usually outlasts photic stimulus
c. Clinical correlate of epilepsy
3. Photomyoclonic response
a. Brief muscle jerks (frontalis, orbicularis oculi), time locked to stimulus frequency
b. No clinical correlate of epilepsy

ABNORMAL EEG PATTERNS

I. Diffuse lesions
   A. Rhythmic slowing
   B. Occasionally periodic discharges
II. Focal lesions
   A. Polymorphic, arrhythmic, unreactive delta
   B. Periodic lateralized epileptiform discharges (PLEDs)
III. Epilepsy
   A. Initial interictal EEG is abnormal in 50%
   B. With repeated recordings, 90–95% will show abnormalities
   C. 2% of normal population have abnormalities considered to be epileptiform
   D. Absence seizures
      1. 3/s spike and wave
      2. 4/s spike and wave in juvenile
      3. Myoclonic absence of Janz response
      4. 2–2.5/s spike and wave in atypical absence
   E. Primary generalized tonic-clonic seizures
      1. Interictal: bursts of spike and wave
      2. Ictal: 10 Hz fast activity during tonic phase, followed by lower frequency spike and wave complexes during clonic phase
      3. Postictal: generalized slowing, delta range
   F. Myoclonic epilepsy
      1. Polyspike and wave
   G. Partial (focal) epilepsy
      1. Interictal: focal spikes or sharp waves
      2. Ictal: focal rhythmic discharge
IV. Periodic complexes
   A. Herpes simplex encephalitis
   B. Creutzfeldt-Jakob disease
   C. Subacute sclerosing panencephalitis

ABNORMAL EEG PATTERNS (*Continued*)

   V. Triphasic waves
      A. Liver, renal, hypoxia or other metabolic encephalopathies
  VI. Frontal intermittent rhythmic delta activity (FIRDA)
      A. Metabolic encephalopathy
 VII. Alpha coma
      A. Widespread, nonreactive alpha-range activity
      B. Severe, generalized encephalopathy
VIII. Burst-suppression
      A. High-voltage bursts, followed by periods of extreme suppression
      B. Severe bihemispheric insult
  IX. Brain death
      A. Minimum 30-minute recording time
      B. Double-distance montage
      C. Low-frequency filter settings below 1 Hz, record at maximal gain
         (2 μV/mm sensitivity), stimulate patient
      D. Hypotension, hypothermia, hypoxia and sedative drug overdose
         must all be excluded

ELECTROMYOGRAPHY

I. Insertional activity
  A. Increased
    1. Normal variant
    2. Denervated muscle
    3. Myotonic disorders
  B. Decreased
    1. Periodic paralysis
    2. Muscle replacement by fat, connective tissue

II. Fibrillation potentials
  A. Lower motor neuron
    1. Anterior horn cell diseases
    2. Polyradiculopathies
    3. Plexopathies
    4. Axonal peripheral neuropathy
    5. Mononeuropathies
  B. Neuromuscular junction
    1. Severe myasthenia gravis
    2. Botulism
  C. Muscle
    1. Myositis
    2. Myotonic dystrophy
    3. Duchenne-type dystrophy
    4. Centronuclear (myotubular) myopathy
    5. Nemaline rod myopathy
    6. Hyperkalemic/normokalemic periodic paralysis
    7. Acid maltase deficiency (type II, Pompe's disease)
    8. Rhabdomyolysis
    9. Trichinosis
    10. Trauma

III. Fasciculations
  A. Normal
    1. Benign fatigue
    2. Benign with cramps
  B. Lower motor neuron disease
    1. Amyotrophic lateral sclerosis
    2. Creutzfeldt-Jakob disease
    3. Nerve root compression
    4. Peripheral neuropathy

ELECTROMYOGRAPHY (*Continued*)

   C. Metabolic
      1. Tetany
      2. Thyrotoxicosis
      3. Cholinesterase inhibitors
 IV. Complex repetitive discharges
   A. Myopathies
      1. Polymyositis/dermatomyositis
      2. Duchenne-type dystrophy
      3. Limb-girdle dystrophy
      4. Hypothyroidism
      5. Glycogen storage diseases
      6. Myotonic chondrodystrophy (Schwartz-Jampel syndrome)
   B. Neurogenic
      1. Spinal muscular atrophy
      2. Poliomyelitis
      3. Amyotrophic lateral sclerosis
      4. Chronic radioculopathy
      5. Charcot-Marie-Tooth disease
      6. Chronic neuropathy
  V. Myotonia
   A. Hyperkalemic/normokalemic periodic paralysis
   B. Myotonic dystrophy
   C. Myotonia congenita of Thomsen
   D. Hypothyroidism
   E. Myotonic chondrodystrophy (Schwartz-Jampel syndrome)
   F. Diazocholesterol
   G. Aromatic amino acids
   H. Clofibrate
    I. Paramyotonia congenita (Eulenburg's disease)
   J. Isaacs syndrome
   K. Acid maltase deficiency (type II, Pompe's disease)
   L. Polymyositis/dermatomyositis
 VI. Myokymia
   A. Facial
      1. Multiple sclerosis
      2. Brainstem glioma
      3. Facial palsy
      4. Polyradiculopathy(?)

List Continues

ELECTROMYOGRAPHY (*Continued*)

    B. Extremity
        1. Radiation plexopathy
        2. Chronic nerve entrapment
VII. Neuromyotonia
    A. Syndrome of continuous muscle fiber activity
    B. Cholinesterase inhibitors
    C. Tetany
    D. Spinal muscular atrophy
VIII. Tetany
    A. Tetanus
    B. Isaacs syndrome
    C. Hypocalcemia
    D. Hypomagnesemia
    E. Water intoxication
    F. Hyperventilation and others
  IX. Cramp potential
    A. Salt depletion
    B. Chronic neurogenic atrophy
    C. Benign nocturnal cramps
    D. Hypothyroidism
    E. Pregnancy
    F. Uremia (dialysis)

MYOGLOBINURIA

I. Hereditary
   A. Myophosphorylase deficiency (type V, McArdle's disease)
   B. Phosphofructokinase deficiency (type VII, Tarui's disease)
   C. Phosphoglycerate kinase deficiency
   D. Phosphoglycerate mutase deficiency
   E. Lactate dehydrogenase deficiency
   F. Carnitine palmityl transferase deficiency
   G. Malignant hyperthermia
   H. Recurrent attacks secondary infection, exercise or spontaneous; defect unknown
II. Sporadic
   A. Exertion (vigorous exercise, anterior tibial syndrome, convulsions, electric shock, tetanus, dystonia, catatonic rigidity, delirium tremens)
   B. Trauma (crush, prolonged coma, ischemia, air embolism, burns)
   C. Metabolic/toxic
      1. Barbiturates, carbon monoxide, narcotic coma
      2. Diabetic ketoacidosis
      3. General anesthesia
      4. Succinylcholine
      5. Amphotericin B
      6. Chronic hypokalemia
      7. Hypophosphatemia
      8. Heroin
      9. Malignant neuroleptic syndrome
      10. Alcoholism
      11. Myotoxic snake bite
      12. Food poisoning (Mediterranean quail, Haff disease)
   D. Heat stroke, hypothermia
   E. Toxic shock syndrome, gram-negative septicemia, leptospirosis
   F. Progressive myopathy (polymyositis, alcoholic myopathy)

BEADING OR SEGMENTAL NARROWING/DILATION OF BLOOD VESSELS

I. Vascular
   A. Arteriosclerosis
   B. Migraine
   C. Fibromuscular dysplasia
   D. Cerebral postpartum angiopathy
   E. Granulomatous angiitis
   F. Lymphomatoid granulomatosis
   G. Hypertensive encephalopathy (in rats)
   H. Moyamoya disease
   I. Primary arterial occlusive diseases in children
   J. Benign distal intracranial arteritis
   K. Carotid arteritis of childhood
   L. Hypersensitivity angiitis
   M. Polyarteritis nodosa
   N. Rheumatoid arthritis
   O. Scleroderma
   P. Systemic lupus erythematosus
   Q. Sickle-cell anemia
   R. Subarachnoid hemorrhage with spasm
   S. Systemic necrotizing vasculitis
   T. Temporal arteritis with intracranial involvement
   U. Wegener's granulomatosis
   V. Dego's disease (malignant atrophic papulosis)

II. Metabolic
   A. Lipoprotein abnormalities
   B. Acromegaly
   C. Toxins

III. Infectious
   A. Purulent meningitis
   B. Tuberculous meningitis
   C. Brain abscess, chronic
   D. Syphilis
   E. Cryptococcosis
   F. Actinoycosis
   G. Herpes zoster ophthalmicus
   H. Cat-scratch disease
   I. Nocardiosis
   J. Sarcoidosis

BEADING OR SEGMENTAL NARROWING/DILATION
OF BLOOD VESSELS (*Continued*)

IV. (Para)neoplastic
- A. Hodgkin's disease
- B. Lymphoma
- C. Metastatic lung cancer
- D. Glioma
- E. Lipoma
- F. Metastatic atrial myxoma
- G. Neoplastic angioendotheliosis
- H. Pheochromocytoma

V. Inherited disorders
- A. Sturge-Weber syndrome
- B. Neurofibromatosis
- C. Tuberous sclerosis

VI. Trauma
- A. Radiation
- B. Surgery (brain)
- C. Miscellaneous trauma

HIGH-DENSITY LESIONS ON CT

I. Blood
   A. Subarachnoid hemorrhage
   B. Subdural hematoma
   C. Epidural hematoma
   D. Brain contusion
   E. Stagnant blood in artery (e.g., middle cerebral artery stem embolus = "string sign")
   F. Intracerebral hemorrhage
   G. Hemorrhage into infarction
   H. Hemorrhage into tumor
   I. Hemorrhage into infected region
   J. Venous thrombosis
II. Calcification
   A. Atherosclerositic blood vessels
   B. Tumor (meningioma, oligodendroglioma, astrocytoma, craniopharyngioma)
   C. Arteriovenous malformation
   D. Hamartoma
   E. Sturge-Weber syndrome
   F. Tuberous sclerosis
   G. Aneurysm
   H. Hamartoma
   I. Pineal gland (normal)
   J. Choroid plexus (normal)
   K. Basal ganglia (may be normal, Fahr's disease, hypoparathyroidism)
   L. Falx (normal)
   M. Scar formation
   N. Infections
      1. Tuberculosis
      2. CMV
      3. Cysts (eg., cysticercosis)
III. Elevated protein
   A. Mucinous adenocarcinoma

LOW-DENSITY LESIONS ON CT

    I. Infarction
   II. Tumor
  III. Abscess
  IV. Edema
    V. Encephalitis
  VI. Resolving hematoma
 VII. Arachnoid cyst
VIII. Lipoma
  IX. Air (after trauma or neurosurgery)
   X. Hydrocephalus/syrinx

LESIONS BY ANATOMICAL LOCATION
(ON CT OR MRI)

I. Pineal region masses
    A. Pineal parenchyma
        1. Pineocytoma
        2. Pineoblastoma
    B. Germ cell
        1. Germinoma
        2. Choriocarcinoma
        3. Teratoma
        4. Teratocarcinoma
        5. Embryonal carcinoma
        6. Dermoid cyst
        7. Epidermoid cyst
    C. Supporting tissues
        1. Astrocytoma
        2. Ependymoma
        3. Meningioma
        4. Cysts
        5. Lipoma
    D. Other
        1. Vein of Galen aneurysm
        2. Glioma of brainstem
        3. Glioma of thalamus
        4. Subsplenial meningioma
        5. Sarcoid granuloma
II. Suprasellar masses
    A. Pituitary adenoma
    B. Meningioma
    C. Metastases
    D. Aneurysm (internal carotid, anterior communicating, basilar tip)
    E. Craniopharyngioma
    F. Optic glioma
    G. Arachnoid cyst
    H. Teratoma
    J. Dermoid cyst
    J. Pineal region tumor (see above)
    K. Hypothalamic glioma
    L. Sarcoid granuloma
    M. Histiocytosis X

LESIONS BY ANATOMICAL LOCATION
(ON CT OR MRI) (*Continued*)

III. Posterior fossa masses
   A. Extra-axial
      1. Foramen magnum
         a. Meningioma
         b. Chordoma
         c. Neurofibroma
      2. Cerebellopontine angle
         a. Acoustic neuroma
         b. Meningioma
         c. Metastases
         d. Vascular malformation
         e. Epidermoid cyst
         f. Exophytic brainstem glioma
         g. Arachnoid cyst
         h. Aneurysm
         i. Choroid plexus papilloma
         j. Chordoma
         k. Trigeminal neuroma
         l. Seventh nerve neuroma
         m. Glomus jugulare tumor
         n. Sarcoid granuloma
   B. Intra-axial
      1. Anterior compartment
         a. Brainstem glioma
         b. Syringobulbia
         c. Cavernous angioma
      2. Posterior compartment (cerebellum)
         a. Metastases
         b. Hemangioblastoma
         c. Cerebellar astrocytoma
         d. Ependymoma
         e. Medulloblastoma
         f. Choroid plexus papilloma
         g. Oligodendroglioma
         h. Ganglioglioma

List Continues

LESIONS BY ANATOMICAL LOCATION
(ON CT OR MRI) (*Continued*)

IV. Spinal cord masses
    A. Intramedullary
        1. Ependymoma
        2. Astrocytoma
        3. Hemangioblastoma
        4. AVM
        5. Hematoma/hematomyelia
        6. Cyst
        7. Syringo/hydromyelia
        8. Cord edema
        9. Lipoma
        10. Abscess
    B. Intradural, extramedullary
        1. Meningioma
        2. Neurofibroma
        3. Metastases
        4. Exophytic ependymoma
        5. Arachnoid cyst
        6. AVM
        7. Hematoma
        8. Lipoma
        9. Dermoid/epidermoid
        10. Subdural hematoma/empyema
    C. Extradural, extramedullary
        1. Metastases (lung, breast, prostate)
        2. Myeloma
        3. Lymphoma
        4. Neurofibroma

LESIONS BY ANATOMICAL LOCATION
(ON CT OR MRI) (*Continued*)

    5. Disc herniation
    6. Vertebral body compression
    7. Trauma (leading to boney fracture, dislocation)
    8. Abscess
    9. TB granuloma
  10. Extramedullary hematopoiesis
  11. Vertebral body expansion (e.g., Paget's disease, hemangioma)
  12. Osteophytes
  13. Spinal stenosis
  14. Hematoma
  15. Lipoma
V. Third ventricular masses
  A. Ependymoma
  B. Teratoma
  C. Meningioma
  D. Parasytic cyst (e.g., cysticercosis)
  E. Glioma
  F. Epidermoid tumor
  G. Dysgerminoma (usually inferior)
  H. Colloid cysts (usually superior/anterior)
  I. Intraventricular meningiomas
  J. Choroid plexus tumors
  K. Granulomas
  L. Arteriovenous malformation
  M. Tubers (hyperplastic nodules seen in tuberous sclerosis)
  N. Neurofibromas

10
MISCELLANEOUS LISTS

SYNDROME OF INAPPROPRIATE ANTIDIURETIC HORMONE (SIADH)

I. CNS
- A. Increased intracranial pressure
- B. Subarachnoid hemorrhage
- C. Subdural hematoma
- D. Brain tumor
- E. Cerebral thrombosis
- F. Head trauma
- G. Central pontine myelinosis

II. Drugs
- A. Carbamazepine
- B. Barbiturates
- C. Chlorpropamide
- D. Clofibrate
- E. Cyclophosphamide
- F. Morphine
- G. Tricyclic antidepressants
- H. Vinblastine
- I. Vincristine
- J. General anesthesia

III. Infection
- A. Meningitis
- B. Encephalitis
- C. Abscess

IV. Tumor
- A. Bronchogenic carcinoma
- B. Adenocarcinoma of the pancreas
- C. Lymphosarcoma

V. Miscellaneous
- A. Guillain-Barré syndrome
- B. Sarcoidosis
- C. Postsurgery
- D. Postpartum

DIABETES INSIPIDUS

   I. Autoimmune
  II. Brain death
 III. Degenerative disease
 IV. Familial
  V. Granulomatous disease
     A. Sarcoidosis
     B. Tuberculosis
     C. Meningovascular syphilis
     D. Wegener's granulomatosis
 VI. Hypoxia
VII. Vascular
     A. Aneurysm of circle of Willis
     B. Subarachnoid hemorrhage
     C. Sheehan syndrome (postpartum pituitary necrosis)
VIII. Idiopathic
 IX. Infection
     A. Abscess
     B. Meningitis
     C. Encephalitis
  X. Radiation
 XI. Malformations
XII. Trauma
     A. Basilar skull fracture through sella turcica
     B. Postoperative (neurosurgical)
XIII. Tumors
     A. Craniopharyngioma
     B. Pituitary adenoma
     C. Meningioma
     D. Optic glioma
     E. Histiocytosis X
     F. Leukemia

AREAS OF THE CNS WITHOUT A BLOOD-BRAIN BARRIER

   I. Pineal body
  II. Subfornical organ
 III. Organum vasculosum of the lamina terminalis (or supraoptic crest)
  IV. Median eminence
   V. Neurohypophysis
  VI. Area postrema
 VII. Olfactory tract
VIII. Choroid plexus (does not have a blood-brain barrier per se, but has a barrier at the level of the cuboidal cells)

SLEEP DISORDERS CLASSIFICATION

I. DIMS: disorders of initiating and maintaining sleep (insomnias)
   A. Psychophysiological
   B. Associated with psychiatric disorders
   C. Associated with use of drugs and alcohol
   D. Associated with sleep-induced respiratory impairment
      1. Sleep apnea
         a. Central, obstructuve, mixed (see separate list)
      2. Alveolar hypoventilation
   E. Periodic movements during sleep
      1. Nocturnal myoclonus
      2. Restless legs syndrome
   F. Associated with other medical, toxic, or environmental conditions
II. DOES: disorders of excessive sleep (hypersomnias)
   A. Psychophysiological
   B. Associated with psychiatric disorders
   C. Associated with use of drugs and alcohol
   D. Associated with sleep-induced respiratory impairment
      1. Sleep apnea
         a. Central, obstructive, mixed (see separate list)
      2. Alveolar hypoventilation
   E. Periodic movements during sleep
      1. Nocturnal myoclonus
      2. Restless legs syndrome
   F. Narcolepsy
   G. Idiopathic CNS hypersomnolence
   H. Intermittent syndromes
      1. Kleine-Levin syndrome
      2. Menstrual associated
   I. Associated with other medical, toxic, or environmental conditions
      (e.g., hepatic/renal failure, hypothyroidism, COPD, hypoglycemia,
      hydrocephalitis, encephalitis, third ventricular lesions)

SLEEP DISORDERS CLASSIFICATION (*Continued*)

III. Dysfunctions associated with sleep, sleep stages, or partial arousals (parasomnias)
- A. Sleepwalking (somnambulism)
- B. Sleep terror (pavor nocturnus, incubus)
- C. Sleep-related enuresis
- D. Other sleep-related dysfunction
  1. Nightmares
  2. Seizures
  3. Bruxism
  4. Headbanging
  5. Familial sleep paralysis
  6. Asthma
  7. Reflux
  8. Paroxysmal nocturnal hemoglobinuria

IV. Disorders of sleep-wake schedule
- A. Jet lag
- B. Shift change
- C. Other persistent alterations in sleep-wake patterns
  1. Delayed sleep phase syndrome
  2. Advanced sleep phase syndrome

SLEEP APNEA SYNDROMES

I. Central
   A. Idiopathic
   B. Physiological
      1. High altitude
      2. Severe hypoxemia
   C. Vascular
      1. Brainstem infarction (e.g., Wallenberg syndrome)
   D. Structural
      1. Neoplasm
      2. Syringobulbia
   E. Infectious
      1. Brainstem encephalitis
      2. Western equine encephalitis
      3. Subacute sclerosing panencephalitis
      4. Postencephalitic parkinsonism
   F. Neurodegenerative
      1. Progressive supranuclear palsy
      2. Alzheimer's disease
      3. Creutzfeldt-Jakob disease
      4. Olivopontocerebellar atrophy
      5. Olivodentate degeneration
      6. Shy-Drager syndrome
II. With narcoplepsy (10–15%)

SLEEP APNEA SYNDROMES (*Continued*)

III. Following high bilateral cordotomies
IV. Nerve lesions
    A. Motor neuron disease
    B. Myasthenia gravis
    C. Guillain-Barré syndrome
  V. Mixed
    A. Autonomic neuropathy
    B. Polycythemia
    C. Down syndrome
VI. Obstructive
    A. Obesity
    B. Adenotonsillar hypertrophy
    C. Acromegaly
    D. Myxedema
    E. Myotonic dystrophy
    F. Thomsen's disease
    G. Deformities of the chest wall
    H. Micrognathia
    I. Möbius, Pierre Robin, Kearns-Sayre, Treacher Collins, Prader-Willi syndromes

(From Critchley EMR: Neurological Emergencies. WB Saunders, London, 1988, with permission.)

INTRANEURONAL INCLUSION BODIES

I. Lewy bodies
  A. Found in idiopathic Parkinson's and Alzheimer's diseases
  B. Progressive autonomic failure
  C. Round concentric hyaline inclusion
  D. Especially in pigmented nuclei
  E. Central mass of filaments and granules
  F. Less dense at periphery of radiating fibers
II. Lafora bodies
  A. Cytoplasmic inclusion
  B. Seen in myoclonic epilepsy, advancing age, and axonal degeneration
  C. Seen in pigmented nuclei, especially dentate
  D. Rounded/concentric
    1. Basophilic core
    2. Peripheral, paler rim
III. Negri bodies
  A. Intracytoplasmic eosinophilic inclusion bodies
  B. Especially in pyramidal cells of the hippocampus
  C. Seen in rabies
IV. Viral inclusion bodies (Cowdry's type A)
  A. Intranuclear (neuron or glia) eosinophilic
  B. Clear halo
  C. Seen in the following:
    1. Poliomyelitis
    2. Herpes
    3. Subacute sclerosing panencephalitis

INTRANEURONAL INCLUSION BODIES (*Continued*)

V. Neurofibrillary tangle
   A. Within cytoplasm
   B. Demonstrated by silver impregnation
   C. Thick black bands
   D. Paired filaments wound in helical fashion
   E. Seen in the following:
      1. Alzheimer's disease
      2. Postencephalitic parkinsonism
      3. Progressive supranuclear palsy (straight filaments)
      4. Guamanian Parkinson-dementia complex
      5. Cerebral cortex of boxers ("dementia pugilistica")
      6. Adult Down syndrome
      7. Aluminum (argyrophilic tangles, but single filaments)

VI. Torpedo
   A. Axonal lesion found in Purkinje cells
   B. Seen well with silver impregnations
   C. Found in systemic degenerations
      1. Olivopontocerebellar atrophy
      2. Vitamin E deficiency
      3. Neuroaxonal dystrophy

VII. Hirano bodies
   A. Short, rod-shaped eosinophilic material
   B. Found in Sommer's sector of hippocampus
   C. Seen in advancing age, Alzheimer's and Pick's diseases
   D. Guamanian Parkinson-dementia complex

ROSENTHAL FIBERS

I. Found in perikarya and processes of astrocytes
   A. Homogeneous, hyaline, eosinophilic structures
   B. Round, oval, or elongated
   C. Variable size (10–40 μm)
   D. Stable to fixation
   E. Granular center
   F. Glial fibrils in periphery
II. Found in long-standing intense fibrillary gliosis
   A. Around syringomyelic cavities or tumors
   B. Slow-growing astrocytomas (especially cerebellum or optic nerve)
   C. Alexander's disease
   D. ?Relation to nickel (reported with nickel electrodes)

Index

Page numbers followed by f indicate figures.